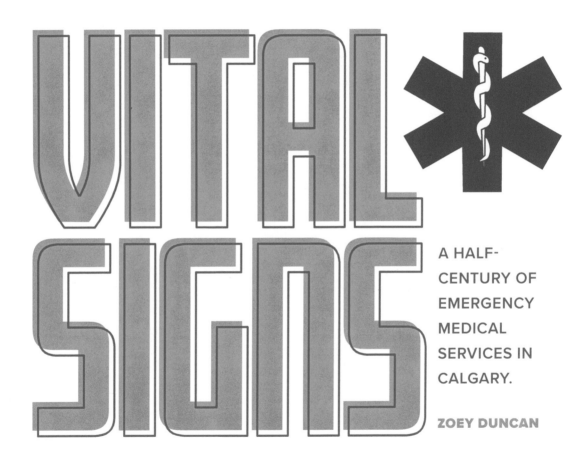

VITAL SIGNS

A HALF-CENTURY OF EMERGENCY MEDICAL SERVICES IN CALGARY.

ZOEY DUNCAN

Published by the Emergency Medical Service (EMS) Foundation
#70, 2626 Country Hills Blvd NE
Calgary, Alberta T3N 1A7

Written by Zoey Duncan
ZoeyDuncan.ca

Proofing by Catherine Szabo

Additional Editing by Tim Prieur, EMS Foundation

Designed by Crystal Ink
crystalink.ca

First Published in 2019

Copyright © Emergency Medical Service (EMS) Foundation, 2019

All rights are reserved. Without limiting the rights under copyright reserved above, no part of this publication may be reproduced, stored or introduced into a retrieval system, or transmitted in any form or by any means (electronic, mechanical, photocopying, recording, or otherwise) without the prior written permission of both the copyright owner and the above publisher of the book.

ISBN 978-1-77136-732-5

Visit the Emergency Medical Service (EMS) Foundation at **emsfoundation.ca**.

In recognition of those individuals
who advanced the delivery of
pre-hospital medical care to the
citizens of Calgary.

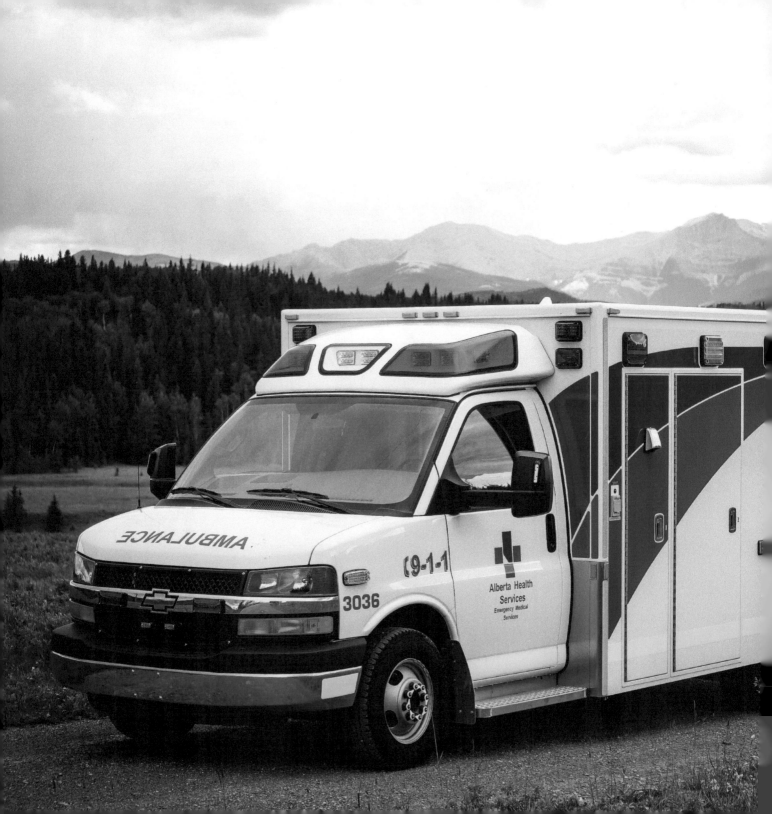

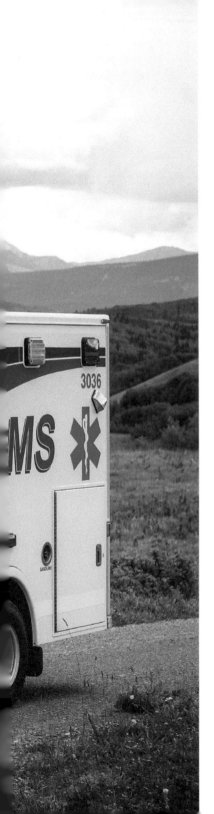

FOREWORD

By Chris Salmon, EMS Foundation Chair

I lay there on the side of the road bleeding. I had just extracted myself from my upside-down car. My thinking was fuzzy. I had glass embedded in my face and hand. A nasty cut to the top of my head that later required some 13 staples to close. No idea how I got out of the vehicle. I remembered that my father had died in a car accident. I was worried about how my family would take the news.

Then I heard the siren. Until that day I had spent time around paramedics as an outsider, working hard to help and support them. Now, I needed their help.

The Emergency Medical Services Foundation is the oldest of its kind in Canada, founded in 1995 by Tom Sampson, then-Chief, EMS, at the City of Calgary. I joined the board of the EMS Foundation in 2015 and was elected board chair in 2016. With the help of a dedicated, passionate, diverse and able team, we have worked hard to make sure our programs support the work of Alberta's paramedics. We do this in three ways:

- supporting new initiatives and research,
- supporting community education and outreach, and,
- preserving the history of paramedicine in Alberta.

The challenging thing about history is that you seldom remember you are living it until it is too late. Behind the uniform you will uncover a rich narrative tapestry of diverse stories and shared experiences that make the listener chuckle or tear up, both in short order.

This book is an attempt to capture some of those stories, lest they are lost to time. I'd like to give a huge thank you to all of the paramedics, active and retired, who gave their time and recollections that made this book possible. A very special thank-you goes to Zoey Duncan for helping us capture and collate those stories.

The Foundation could not exist without the support of a number of key stakeholders. I would like to thank AHS Paramedic Chief Darren Sandbeck, EMS executive directors Nicolas Thain, Dale Weiss and Marty Scott, Alberta Health Services CEO Dr. Verna Yiu, City of Calgary Director Christine Arthurs, Alberta College of Paramedics President Pete Helfrich, CEMA Chief Tom Sampson, HSAA President Mike Parker and the board of the EMS Foundation.

While the story of how we got here has many players, I'd particularly like to thank the contributions of Brent Foster, Dr. Tim Prieur, Kim McCulley, Adam Loria, Stuart Brideaux, Lisa Barrett, Ashley McKay, Jared Hendry, Ed Chamberlain, Jordie Frasier, Nathanial Pike, Dell Harrison, Alex Campbell, Daphne Stevenson and Kayla Primiani. Without your help the Foundation could not function. Thank you.

Finally, I would like to thank the paramedics of Alberta, whether Alberta Health Services EMS or contracted. Every day you make a difference. Thank you.

To the paramedic who helped me in that ditch at 5 a.m. in May 2017. Thank you.

CONTENTS

The Private Ambulance Era
Pre-1971

— 1 —

The Calgary Fire Department Era
1971-1984

— 25 —

The New Boomtown Era
1984-1994

— 61 —

The Hallway Medic Era
1994-2009

— 83 —

The Provincial Health Care Era
2009-2019

— 105 —

Never Forgotten

— 125 —

THE PRIVATE AMBULANCE ERA
PRE-1971

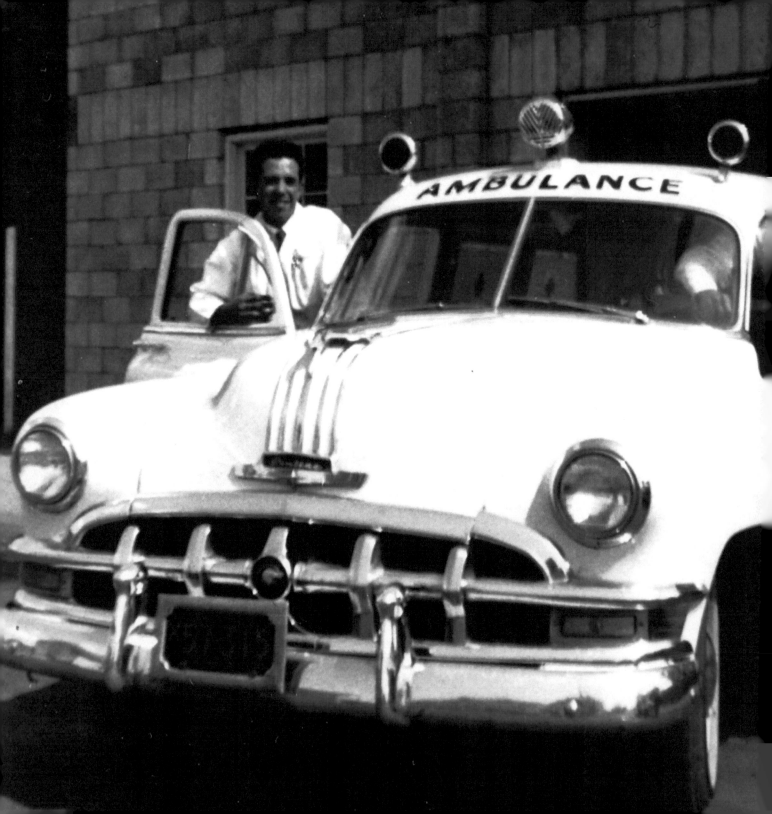

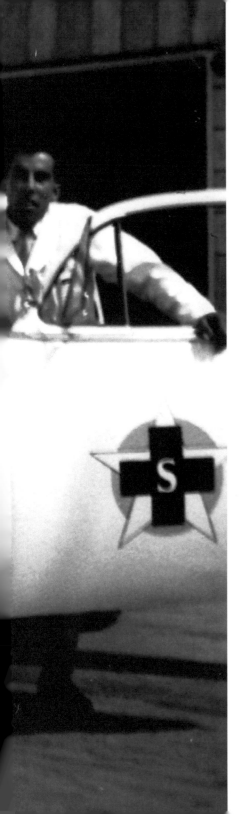

FIRST AID AND FISTICUFFS

Let's set the scene. It's the early 1960s and Alberta's second-largest city is home to about 270,000 people. The most recognizable feature of the city's young skyline is the Calgary General Hospital on the shores of the Bow River. Agriculture is a big driver of economic activity in Calgary and Alberta, but the petroleum extraction industry is beginning to build steam, thanks to some oil found up north about 15 years earlier. Nobody knows yet the oil discovery was the start of something that would change the city forever, bringing a million more people (and potential patients) to Calgary over the next half-century.

It was a time before mandatory seatbelts, safety goggles and steel-toed boots. But at the same time, there were human experiences happening then that haven't changed. People still delivered babies, suffered traumatic accidents and had medical emergencies. And for those moments and many more unpredictable situations where life and limb were at risk, Calgary's private ambulance companies were there to help as best they could.

For early ambulance companies, like Starr's Ambulance pictured here in the 1950s, horizontal transportation from point A to point B was the best medical service they could provide. (Courtesy of Gary Fisher)

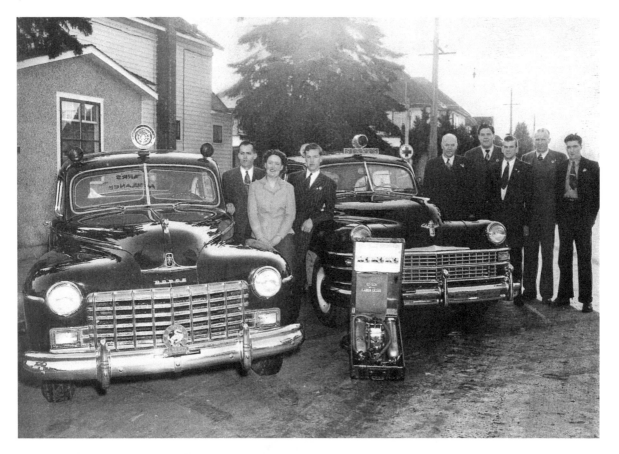

Staff from Starr's Ambulance in the late 1940s, including Rose Skopdepo, Gerry Price, Bryan Hart, Bill Hill, Dave Coulter and Homer Rodgers. (Courtesy of Gary Fisher)

The earliest ambulance services in Calgary were provided by funeral homes. As in many towns and cities in the early part of the 20th century, the funeral homes' hearses—first horse-drawn wagons, then later cars—transported patients to hospital. The carts and cars had no blood-mopping, wound-cleaning or life-saving equipment onboard, nor did their drivers have first-aid training, but it was still the best way to get to a doctor in an emergency. By the 1930s, a handful of ambulance companies operated out of service garages or their own dedicated stations, and that's when competition started to heat up.

THE PRIVATE AMBULANCE ERA PRE-1971

Perhaps the best way to illustrate Calgary's private ambulance industry in the '60s is to paint a picture of what a motor vehicle collision scene may have looked like. The first ambulance to arrive on scene could have been Universal Ambulance, with a two-man crew arriving in a custom Chevrolet ambulance. Hot on the scene right after them is a Starr's Ambulance crew in a cherry-red custom Cadillac ambulance. One of these ambulance companies has a contract with the City, making them the sole operator to provide emergency ambulance service. The City contract paid roughly $50,000 for three years of emergency ambulance services. This was a pretty good contract, at least until the figure was no longer sufficient to cover the real costs of ambulance services in a growing city.

The ambulance companies without the City contract used a police radio to monitor for injury reports. Technically, it was illegal to use a police radio for business purposes, so the strategy was to not keep the police radio at ambulance stations. Whoever's job it was to listen to the radio would call in accidents to the station, and an ambulance was dispatched. Sometimes they beat the competition there, scooped their patient up and sped off to the hospital. But other times, arriving on scene was where the trouble began.

Cars like this 1953 Eureka Cadillac ambulance from Associated Ambulance's fleet would have been a joy to drive. (Courtesy of Fred Underhill)

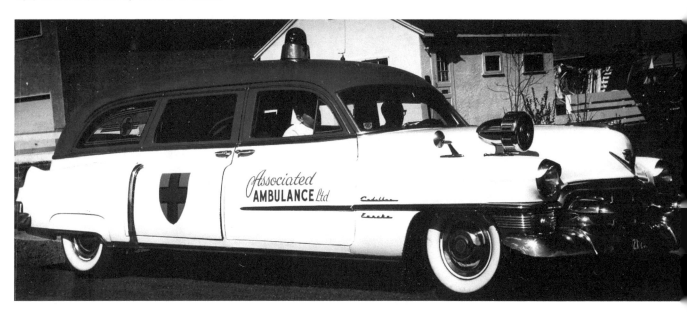

It wasn't unusual for rival ambulance companies to fight over patients in all senses of the word. Battles for patients tended to be rooted in a desire to get paid, not necessarily a desire to help the patient the most. Ambulance companies relied on patients' insurance companies paying their ambulance bills so they could pay their attendants and drivers. In the small city of Calgary, there were only so many ambulance trips to go around. This fierce competition manifested in a variety of creative, nefarious and at-times downright shocking ways, both at the scene and beyond. For example, the second ambulance crew to arrive on scene might see the first crew had already loaded their patient into the back of the ambulance and had set off attending to another potential patient. Well, that's a convenient opportunity for the second crew to extract the patient and load them into their own ambulance. Or perhaps the second crew would park their vehicle such that the back of the first ambulance was inaccessible. Or maybe an ambulance mysteriously developed a flat tire. Ambulances were left running at the scene, with their lights flashing and the keys in the ignition, so a rival "ambulance man" might remove those keys and toss them in a ditch. There was at least one tale of an employee entering a rival company's garage and pouring sugar in the gas tank. It not only took the ambulance off the road for a while, it cost a pretty penny to replace the engine. It's no surprise, then, that fistfights and shouting matches occasionally accompanied some scenes. It wasn't a good look.

There were plenty of days when ambulance attendants were able to execute their roles without altercation. The primary goal of the ambulance attendants of the day was timely transport to hospital. Both the driver (who was the senior crew member, because those custom ambulances were precious) and the attendant were required to have a St. John's Ambulance First Aid Certificate, awarded after the completion of a 14-hour course. Ideally, they'd both have a Class 4 driver's licence, too. In practice, this meant that while they may be able to help stabilize the patient in the field, the best bet for the patient would come from getting them to the hospital as quickly as possible. They didn't have the training or supplies to do much more than that. "You could pretty much just give them oxygen and make them feel comfortable," said Gary Fisher, who worked in the era.

"It was glorified first aid, really," said Ron Firth, who later became a superintendent in EMS.

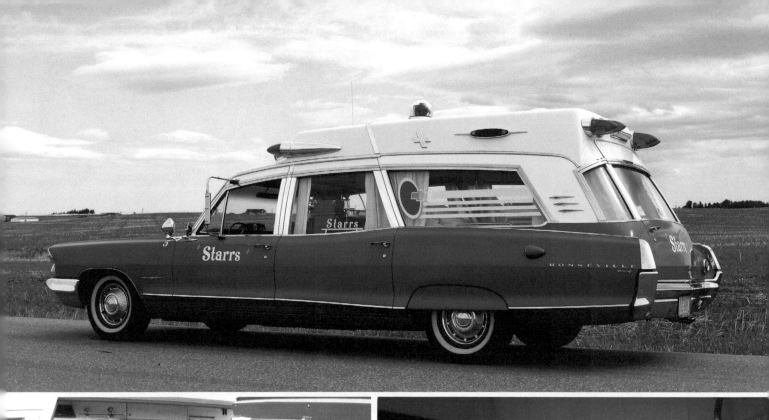
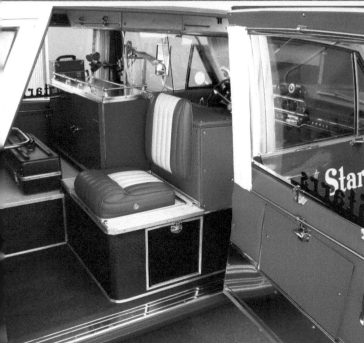
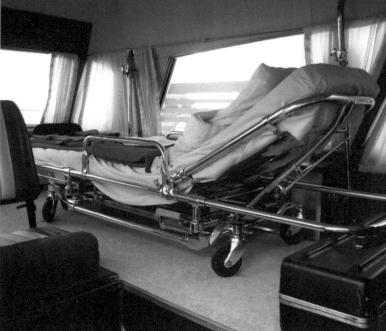

All of Starr's Ambulance's cars were run into the ground thanks to a high workload. This vehicle is an identical sister car to the 1965 Superior Pontiac operated by Starr's. If necessary, up to four patients on stretchers could fit in the back. (Courtesy of Tim Prieur)

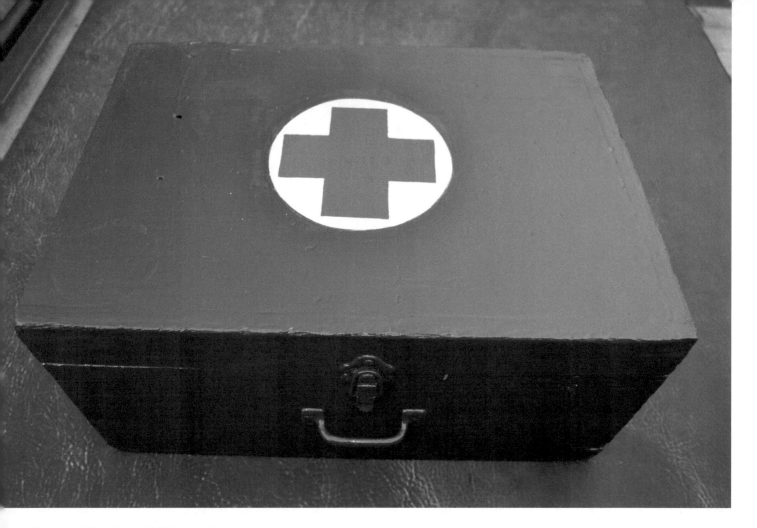

The first aid box from a 1960 Associated Ambulance vehicle held some bandages and gauze, but not much more. (Courtesy of Fred Underhill)

SCOOP AND RUN AND CROSS YOUR FINGERS

Some patients arrived at the hospital in worse condition than they were at the scene. "Treatment was abysmal," said Ron McManus, who went on to become an EMS superintendent. "But it was the best they could do at the time." The technology, training and vehicles to do more just didn't exist yet. It's what paramedics today look back at and call a "scoop and run" service.

THE PRIVATE AMBULANCE ERA PRE-1971

Onboard these ambulances, the crown jewel of equipment was the portable oxygen, which arrived on ambulances in the 1950s. Oxygen was primarily used for treating respiratory concerns and apparent heart attacks, and there was a belief at the time it might help with pain management. Plus, the ambulance company could bill the patient's insurance $6 for its use. Oxygen was the most sophisticated gear onboard for quite some time. Most of what attendants had on hand was more or less the same tools medics had been using since at least the turn of the century. This was partly because ambulance companies tended to have

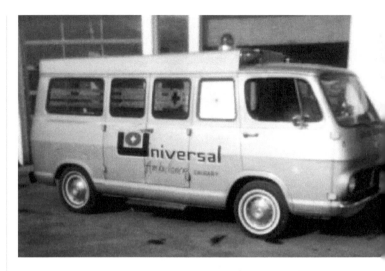

While it was more cost-effective for ambulance companies to build their own vehicles locally, van models were almost universally loathed for their dismal engine power. Gary Fisher recalled driving such a van, with lights and sirens, uphill on 14th Street N.W. and having other drivers pass him by. (Courtesy of Clay Switzer)

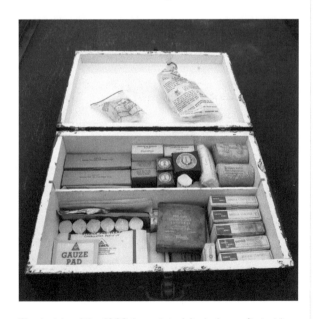

The inside of the 1960 Associated Ambulance first aid box held some bandages and gauze, but not much more. (Courtesy of Fred Underhill)

tight budgets. There was never enough money to do everything they dreamed of.

You could just about count inventory on one hand. An ambulance carried: sterile wound dressings, four-by-four-inch gauze, triangular bandages, airways, wooden splints, a spine board and some freshly laundered linens. Those linens came in handy when a patient had a suspected neck injury. There were no cervical collars onboard (they were too expensive), so those linen sheets were folded up to be about 18 inches long and eight inches thick, wrapped around a patient's neck and secured with a triangular bandage.

9

"WHERE TO BUY IT" — Ambulances—Apartments

A Ambulance
AMhrst 3-2588

FULLY QUALIFIED PERSONNEL

INDUSTRIAL AMBULANCES AVAILABLE ON RENTAL BASIS

A AMBULANCE SERVICE

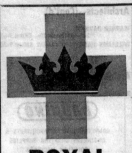

ROYAL AMBULANCE SERVICE
"Calgary's Newest and Finest"

PHONE
CRstvw 7-1333
CRstvw 7-2288

207 - 26th Avenue N.W.

Ambulances
A & A AMBULANCE SERVICE
　1316 Centre St S .. AMhrst 2-1725
A AMBULANCE SERVICE
　216 12 Av SE .. AMhrst 3-2588
　(See Advertisement This Page)
CALGARY AMBULANCE SERVICES LTD
　1316 Centre St S .. AMhrst 2-2636
　(See Advertisement This Page)
ROYAL AMBULANCE SERVICE { CRstvw 7-1333
　207 26 Av NW .... { CRstvw 7-2288
　(See Advertisement This Page)
STAMPEDE AMBULANCE SERVICE
　216 12 Av SE .. AMhrst 3-4210
　(See Advertisement This Page)
STARR'S AMBULANCE SERVICE
　1316 Centre St S .. AMhrst 2-2428
　(See Advertisement This Page)

Antique Dealers
BASHFORDS CORNER LTD
Large Collection of
ANTIQUES & DECORATIVE ACCESSORIES
Imported from Britain, Europe and The Middle East
736 17 Av SW .... AMhrst 9-3560

GENERAL FURNITURE STORE
Antiques of All Kinds Bought and Sold
We Import Cabinet Work to Order
FRENCH POLISHING
UPHOLSTERING
1001 17 Av SW .... CHery 4-2655

Antique Dealers—(Cont'd)
HEIRLOOM ANTIQUE JEWELLERY
Large Collection of
China, Bric-Brac, Clocks and Jewellery
Old Gold, Silver and Coins Bought
GOODS TAKEN ON CONSIGNMENT
346 17 Av SW .... AMhrst 9-2106

SUPERIOR FRENCH POLISHERS
Dan Skibo
Dealers in Antique Furniture
ALL TYPES OF ANTIQUE FURNITURE
BOUGHT, SOLD and REPAIRED
2603 14 St SW .... CHery 4-1548

Apartments Blocks & Buildings
For complete list of Apartments Blocks & Buildings see last page in Yellow Pages Section
Anderson Apartments 18Av&7StSW .. CHery 4-3295
Argyle Court 25ArgyleCrt .... AMhrst 6-4591
Athlone Apartments 7AthloneApts .. AMhrst 2-7882
Burns Building 204BurnsBldg ...... AMhrst 9-3588
Carolina Apartments Hotel
　17-1722 5aStSW .. AMhrst 2-7554
Dahlsen Apartments 5-1030 12AvSW CHery 4-6249
Dawson Apartments 314 6StSW .. AMhrst 6-2691
Devenish Apartments
　112-908 17AvSW .. CHery 4-4950
Dufferin Lodge 517 13AvSW ...... AMhrst 6-4413
Garden Apartment 323a 14AvSW .. AMhrst 2-9263

(Continued Next Page)

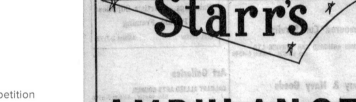

Starr's AMBULANCE
AM2-2428
AM2-2636
CALGARY AMBULANCE SERVICES LTD.
1316 CENTRE STREET S.

STAMPEDE AMBULANCE
AMhrst 3-4210

Radio Dispatched Cars

Six Units Oxygen Equipped

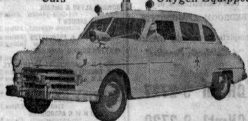

— FULLY QUALIFIED PERSONNEL —
INDUSTRIAL AMBULANCES AVAILABLE ON RENTAL BASIS
STAMPEDE AMBULANCE SERVICE

The competition between ambulance companies was as fierce on the streets as it was in the Yellow Pages, as these pages from 1950 can attest. (Courtesy of Tim Prieur)

"WHERE TO BUY IT"

Aluminum—Consultants
Bassarab R N & Associates Limited
  66EagleRidgeDr..252-6139

Aluminum Doors
See Doors—Metal

Aluminum Fabricators
BARBER MACHINERY CO LIMITED
  4608MacleodTr..243-6061
WEMAS METAL MFG CO LTD
  616 35AvNE..276-4451

Aluminum Siding
See Siding

Aluminum Strapping
See Steel Strapping

Aluminum Windows
See Windows—Metal

LONG DISTANCE
APPOINTMENTS
SAVE TIME AND MONEY
  Avoid wasted trips,
  Allow better planning of your time.
  Make certain you are expected.
  Avoid long delays in waiting to see people.
  Enable your prospects to prepare for your visits.

Ambulance & Hearses Mfrs
SORENSEN DISTRIBUTORS LTD
  4918 52St..Red Deer 346-4812
  G L Sorensen Mgr res....Red Deer 346-2534
Sunnyside Truck Body Industries Ltd
  3619 2StNE..276-4402
SYNTAX CORPORATION OF CANADA
  Mfg Div of Universal Ambulance
  1511 14StSW..244-0777

Ambulances
AARON AMBULANCE & RESUSCITATION
  SERVICE 1347 12AvSW..245-3383
  Accounting Office..................245-1632
  (See Advertisement This Page)
STARR'S AMBULANCE LTD
  1511 14StSW..264-4141
  (See Advertisement This Page)
Sunawagold Kennels Ltd
  Small Animals Only
  5813CrowchildTrNW..............288-5471
UNIVERSAL AMBULANCE SERVICE
  1511 14StSW..245-3333
  Office........................244-0777
  (See Advertisement This Page)

DIAMOND RING LORE
  The diamond, symbol of love, is worn on the fourth finger of the left hand because it was once believed that the vena amoris, or vein of love, ran from this finger directly to the heart. The English Prayer Book of 1549 specified that the marriage ring also be placed on the left hand.

STARR'S
AMBULANCE
SERVICE LTD.

2a-1440a - 17th AVENUE S.W.
ACCOUNTS
244-0779

264-4141

CALGARY'S OLDEST NAME IN AMBULANCE SERVICE

AARON AMBULANCE
245-3383

NEW HEART-LUNG RESUSCITATOR EQUIPPED
24 HOUR SERVICE

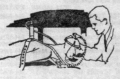

AMBULANCE CHARGES IN ACCORDANCE WITH THE ALBERTA HEALTH PLANS SCHEDULED RATE OF FEES

NO ADDITIONAL CHARGE TO PATIENT
EMERGENCY DOCTORS ON 24 HOUR CALL

AARON AMBULANCE & RESUSCITATION SERVICE
Accounting Office: 1347 - 12th Avenue S.W. 245-1652

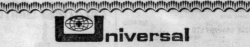

Universal
Ambulance Service

3 LOCATIONS
North   South   West

• Radio and Oxygen Equipped Ambulances

NEW HEART-LUNG RESUSCITATOR
IN-TRANSIT OXYGEN-POWERED EMERGENCY SERVICE
"Dependable Promptness with Safety First"

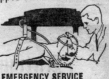

245-3333
24 HOUR SERVICE

OFFICE 1511 - 14th Street S.W. 244-0777
ALBERTA HEALTH PLAN APPROVED

By the late 1960s, some local companies could set themselves apart thanks to their technology, such as heart-lung resuscitators on the vehicles. (Courtesy of Tim Prieur)

If a patient required CPR, which was developed in 1960 following the advent of mouth-to-mouth resuscitation in the mid-1950s, it was initiated without any barrier to protect both parties from germs, a practice that continued until HIV/AIDS arrived in the 1980s. There were no drugs of any kind onboard until after 1971.

By the mid-to-late 1960s, local ambulance companies started to add some higher tech equipment. Universal Ambulance was the first to add a suction unit, both mobile and portable units, for clearing airways. In 1968, the Kiwanis Club donated heart-lung resuscitators to Universal. These predecessors to defibrillators were mechanical CPR units with oxygen tanks, which were game changers when a patient was in cardiac arrest.

With so little equipment to worry about, most ambulances weren't designed to hold much. Many ambulances of the day had minimal headroom because they were customized by ambulance company owners from vans or cars instead of buying expensive models from ambulance suppliers. A single belt-less seat in the back for the attendant was positioned at the patient's head, meaning if the patient required immediate attention to anything lower than their abdomen, the attendant would need to leave their seat and risk getting bounced around the back of the vehicle. Certain high-top ambulances could fit up to four stretcher patients at once, but the hanging-stretcher design allowed only for transport to hospital, rather than any work on the go. Some van conversion ambulances only had a seat up front for the driver, since it was cheaper to forego a passenger seat and instead have the attendant sit in the seat in the back, even when driving without a patient. But the attendant might prefer to sit up front, in which case he'd sit on an upturned metal garbage can with a cushion (probably borrowed from a hospital) on top. It didn't exactly instil confidence for the public to see a paramedic jump out of their ambulance and see an old pail clatter to the ground behind them.

Whichever ambulance company had the City contract also probably had the most ambulances on the road, with four to six serving the population during the day or night. (The competition, on the other hand, would have one or two ambulances on the street.) Ambulance companies might have multiple stations or a single headquarters. A day shift ran from 0800–1800 hours. There were the emergency dispatch calls to deal with, perhaps eight to 10 emergency calls a day, and some chores to be done around the station.

For decades, the city's only two emergency departments were at the Calgary General Hospital and the Holy Cross Hospital, both near downtown. Later in the 1960s, the Rockyview Hospital opened near the south end of the city, followed a few years later by the Foothills Hospital in the far north reaches, each with emergency departments of their own. Emergency departments were staffed by general practitioners who were either interested in what would become known as trauma and emergency medicine or, they just had to do their shift in the emergency room to earn hospital privileges. Without privileges, a doctor can't work out of the hospital or use its resources. Specialization by physicians and surgeons was becoming more common, but Calgary was still decades away from having emergency medicine specialists in its emergency departments.

Patient drop-offs at these emergency departments were quick affairs. Ambulance driver attendants brought their patient in, transferred them onto a hospital bed, and then went on their way in minutes... unless they had time to stop for a cookie or a smoke in the break room and chat with their hospital friends.

It wasn't a terribly hectic job most days. In addition to responding to emergency calls, ambulance companies filled their time with other contracts. Ambulance companies were responsible for transfers between nursing homes and hospitals and for getting patients to the Holy Cross Hospital's cancer clinic. These transfers were organized on a contract basis with individual care homes and hospitals. Starr's also provided residential oxygen tank rental delivery services and had a large supply of oxygen tanks on hand.

After sundown, they'd fulfil their contracts with funeral homes. At Starr's-Associated (the companies merged in 1966), a crew would be dispatched to transfer a deceased patient from the hospital to the appropriate funeral home. That meant picking up the funeral chapel keys from ambulance company headquarters, driving to the hospital to retrieve the deceased, signing out the remains and transporting them to the funeral home. That one was a tough job, retired paramedic Gary Fisher said, particularly when the body being transferred was someone he had been called to help earlier in the day. "You work your butt off trying to save somebody and if you don't, you have to take them to a funeral home." In the late 1970s, a private body removal service took over this role.

Having a dark sense of humour was one way the ambulance staffers approached their work. Retired paramedic Richard Sigurdson said he and his colleagues "would make light of the situation, but not the people involved. You can't take anything that happens out there personally. ... You don't win them all."

The preparation room in a funeral home would invariably be located in the basement with some kind of freight elevator to lower the stretcher and body down. One local funeral home had "a particularly ghoulish elevator," wrote Bill McComb. It was made of wood, painted black, operated by a rope and lit only by a dim bulb. The lights in the basement were always turned off, so an ambulance attendant had to walk a dark hallway to the door of the preparation room and reach inside to locate the light switch.

When an ambulance crew included a rookie on one of their first night shifts, they might have particular trouble with this funeral home. The ambulance with the rookie on board would be given the body removal assignment while another crew would proceed straight to the funeral home, park their ambulance out of sight and set the stage. The rookie's partner might mention how, "a few people over the years have been placed on the slab in the mortuary and were later found to still be alive." In this scenario, one of the stage crew would lie on the slab, covered with a sheet, awaiting the arrival of the new guy. The rookie was told it was his duty to feel his way down the dark hallway and turn on the lights. "It was said that at least one of these unlucky souls fled into the night, never to return to the job," wrote McComb.

Another version of this hazing would have one of the stage crew soak his hand in cold water while awaiting the arrival of the transporting crew. Then he would stand in the dark and wait for the rookie's hand to fumble for the light switch before reaching out and firmly clutching the wrist with a cold and clammy hand. "Guaranteed to cause heart palpitations," wrote McComb.

Dispatch operated under the limitations of technology at the time. The local companies covered an area beyond city limits. Until mobile radios were installed in cars, ambulances were dispatched directly from their stations to the scene of an emergency. There was no reliable way to dispatch them from a mobile location. Occasionally, a shift might get busy, in which case a two-man crew would split up, each driving an ambulance, hopefully with enough time to pick up a temporary partner for an hour. Specifically, they would drive downtown, looking for a police officer walking his beat. Police were pretty easy to find at the time, because most of them walked rather than drove. The ambulance man would tell the officer they needed help at an emergency, then the two would speed off in the ambulance. At the scene, the ambulance man took over the medical concerns and once the patient was loaded in, the police officer drove to the hospital while the attendant stayed with the patient in the back. Or, worst case, if the driver couldn't make a police buddy, he would head to the scene solo and would leave the patient on their own in the back of the ambulance.

One of the universally loathed parts of being an ambulance attendant or driver was bill collection. There was no federal Medicare program until 1966 and few Calgarians had direct billing to their health insurance companies. Many patients were expected to pay their bill directly to the ambulance company. But in the battle between an ambulance staffer writing up receipts or transferring critical patients to emergency rooms, typically the patient's health care won out. Plus, it was awkward for the drivers to try to get a bill paid in a time of crisis for the patient or their family. Over time, that was bad news for ambulance services that relied on those bills ($20 per ride, plus $6 for oxygen, plus $1 per mile) to keep their services running.

By the late 1960s, Blue Cross stopped providing coverage for ambulance rides and it effectively killed Starr's Ambulance. Starr's was so cash-strapped that rather than paying to fix a faulty emergency brake, the crew would carry around a snow shovel. When they parked on a hill, they jammed the shovel under a wheel to keep the ambulance from rolling away. Gary Fisher recalled that if he didn't cash his Starr's paycheque first thing in the morning on payday, there was a risk there'd be no money in the bank by the afternoon. For a long time, bill collection was the main driver for collecting any information about the patient. A patient's name, date of birth, address and insurance information took priority—at least in the receipt book—over recording their illness or injury and what treatment was taken.

In the 1950s, a Calgary ambulance employee made the enticing wage of $1.25 an hour, a pretty good middle-class wage at the time. But as the years passed, wages didn't keep up with inflation or the rising cost of living in Calgary. The job was largely a part-time gig and it was certainly a job, not a career. Some ambulance men loved the thrill of driving fast, or the glory of helping people in dire situations. Some were also transit operators or truck drivers; others were firefighters. With so many part-timers on ambulance services, crews were constantly changing. A two-man crew was lucky if they worked with the same partner two days in a row.

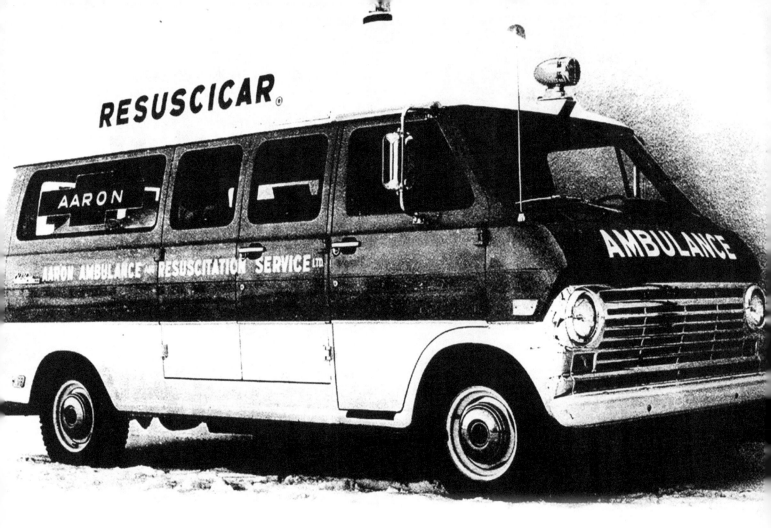

You can drive the emergency room to the patient, but you might not be able to get the emergency room up a hill very quickly. The Aaron Ambulance Resuscicar was ahead of its time in concept. (Courtesy of Tim Prieur)

WE KNEW THE STICKY SIDE WENT DOWN

In the 1960s in Calgary, people within the medical community and the general public were starting to look for ways to improve patients' results after their ambulance ride. A common joke in the job was "Well, we know the sticky side of the bandage goes down." At one local company, a physician thought he could do better than sticky side down. Dr. Peter Cohen, head of the emergency department at the Calgary General Hospital, operated Aaron Ambulance with Richard Sigurdson and Otto Kutsch. Cohen was a pioneer in pre-hospital training, including developing a futuristic mobile emergency room.

Aaron Ambulance operated out of Cohen's clinic. The doctor was born in the Netherlands and wanted to bring the European model for ambulance service to Canada: doctors on every ambulance. It was a great idea in theory. After all, a doctor could do a lot more for a patient—even in the field without much equipment—compared to the first-aid-trained ambulance attendants.

Cohen didn't want to put doctors on a regular ambulance. He wanted them on the Resuscicar. Aaron co-owner Kutsch built the original Resuscicar, then Cohen took it a step further with the version he built out of a Ford van. His goal: to bring the emergency room to the patient. The Resuscicar was a treatment centre first, a transport method second. The ambulance had a raised roof—a necessity considering all the equipment and supplies Cohen was going to put in there. It was like a cross between a motor home and an ambulance. It had hot and cold running water, a heater for blankets, and a huge hydraulic stretcher that could be raised, lowered and angled. The stretcher was modelled on the ones used in an operating room, which made it useful for working on a patient, but hugely impractical for transferring one. It didn't have wheels.

Only the top could be removed—a rectangular frame with cloth stretched across it. In short, not a practical stretcher for most calls. The vehicle also had cutting-edge ambulance technology, including a heart-lung resuscitator and a Lifepak heart monitor. But there were practical limits on what Cohen could do. The Resuscicar was stocked with IV fluids, which came in glass bottles that broke easily. The motor was a real clunker. The Resuscicar struggled to climb hills and, in the words of former Aaron driver Ron McManus, "it handled like a washbowl." Turns had to be navigated carefully, or the whole thing might roll.

Cohen wanted the best people on his ambulance. He couldn't put a doctor on every ambulance. Most doctors didn't want to sit around waiting for calls when they could be seeing (and billing) patients at their office all day. Plus, an ambulance company couldn't afford to pay one doctor, let alone multiple doctors. So Cohen sought to hire nurses and respiratory therapists to join his ambulance attendants and drivers. It was a task easier said than done. He struggled to find enough nurses who were willing to do the physical labour related to ambulance work, like carrying the stretcher and getting dirty in the field (the nurses were more interested in starting IVs and administering medication). And again, he couldn't afford to pay these higher skilled workers on an ambulance company budget.

Ann Sigurdson worked as a nurse in Cohen's office. She recalled one afternoon shortly after she was hired when an ambulance call came in for an injury downtown. All of the other ambulances and staff were out on calls already and there were patients in Cohen's waiting room. Cohen decided he should attend the call. He conscripted a nervous Ann into the Resuscicar. "I was such a nervous wreck," she said, referring partly to Cohen's driving and partly to her lack of training for these situations. The call turned out fine though, and the two of them got back to the office after stabilizing the patient and bringing him to the ER. Ann said it wasn't until much later she learned Cohen saved several lives by attending to certain major trauma calls.

But Cohen's dreams were too big for the resources of the day. "He wanted to do what they're doing today," said Richard Sigurdson. "He was way ahead of his time."

If Cohen couldn't staff his ambulances with people who were highly trained, then he figured at least he could train his people more highly. In 1970, Cohen adapted a training program the U.S. military developed based on their medics' field experience in the Korean and Vietnam wars. Those wars were the first time advanced life support (ALS) was performed in the field. Rather than transport being the priority in battle (getting the wounded back to a hospital), the patient was stabilized as much as possible first before they were moved, including stabilizing spinal injuries, starting IVs and drug administration. A lot more people were making it to the hospital alive than before. The same approach was presumed to be practical in cities, too. Based on the U.S. military program, Cohen ran his lectures at 0600 hours, with the night shift staying late and the day shift coming early to attend. It was the first Canadian emergency medical training program. "We were going to be super trained," said Richard Sigurdson. It was a glimpse of what was to come to Calgary's pre-hospital care in just a few short years.

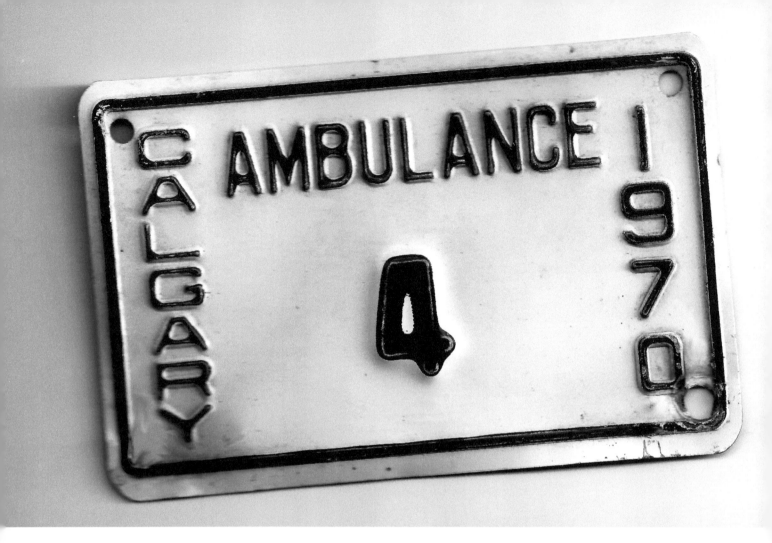

Just as the City of Calgary licenses taxis today, it once licensed ambulances. This particular plate from 1970 was rescued off of an ambulance bound for the crusher. It's believed to be the only one of its kind left. (Courtesy of Tim Prieur)

A STABBING, A STRIKE AND A REPORT

As the decade waned, local doctors were increasingly advocating for pre-hospital medical care to be carried out by ambulance attendants, rather than the scoop and run approach that had been accepted for so long. At the same time, ambulance employees wanted better wages, benefits and career mobility.

In January 1970, Universal Ambulance attendants Lorne Stevens and Dave Jensen were dispatched to a home in Connaught, where an elderly woman had collapsed. They hadn't been told a boy and his mother were also in the home, being held hostage at knifepoint.[1] Stevens and Jensen entered the home, gave the collapsed woman oxygen and loaded her onto a stretcher. That's when a man with a hunting knife, later identified as a boarder in the apartment, threatened them. Stevens told the man they had to get their patient to a hospital, and he seemed to calm down. The woman and her son tried to leave with the ambulance attendants, to accompany the patient and escape a dangerous situation, but the man became angry. He shut the door on Stevens, trapping the mother and boy inside. Stevens pushed the door back open and the man responded by stabbing him in the stomach.

Stevens called the police and drove his bloodied self and Jensen, who was attending to the patient in the back, to the Holy Cross Hospital. While Stevens had surgery, police were able to rescue the woman and her son.

That wasn't the end of the event for Stevens. He planned to go directly to city council to demand better funding for

---

1 Hunter, Mike. "Ambulance Man Stabbed Trying to Rescue Patient." *Albertan* (Calgary), Jan. 23, 1970.

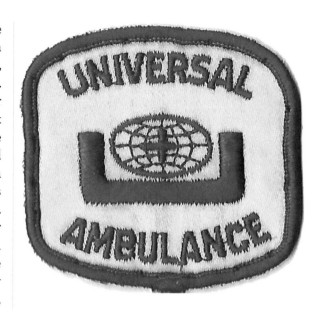

Universal Ambulance shoulder crest.
(Courtesy of Gerry Dilschneider)

ambulance attendants. He told the *Albertan*, "I'll get to that council meeting if I have to on a stretcher. We have to put up with things like this—all for $1.65 an hour." (Minimum wage at the time was $1.25.) "I want to tell council this city gets the best ambulance service in the country for next to nothing." Stevens had previously been held at gunpoint twice and physically assaulted on "several occasions" in his job, according to the *Albertan*.

Stevens' words had an effect. His colleagues at Universal Ambulance, which had the City contract for ambulance service at the time, went on strike in July. For extra impact, they timed it to coincide with the 1970 Calgary

Stampede. They demanded the City fund a wage increase and benefits.

While they were on strike, Aaron Ambulance took over the City contract. With only three ambulances, Aaron wasn't properly equipped to handle the call load and ambulance shortages ensued. "It was crazy!" said paramedic Ron McManus. During the strike, a Universal spokesman told the *Calgary Herald*: "We think we can make more money on welfare than the $1.54 an hour we earned at Universal."[2]

As a result, in November 1970, the Citizens' Emergency Medical Services Advisory Council was created. The advisory council, chaired by Alderman Eric Musgreave, made a report to city council recommending the City take over ambulance service. The report recommended buying out existing ambulance companies and giving the City sole authority for ambulance service.[3] Among its main recommendations were that an emergency medical services division be established within the Calgary Fire Department "separate and distinct from the Fire Fighting service, except for the use of common dispatch and equipment." That separation was notable. Some North American ambulance services at the time were dual-trained services where everyone was trained as both a firefighter and an Emergency Medical Technician. Calgary's proposed service would separate the two distinct groups in rank, while housing them under the same roof. The advisory council perhaps didn't predict this would be a recipe for conflict. It was viewed as a shrewd financial move. The fire department already had stations and systems designed to respond to emergencies, so setting up the ambulance service there seemed the most practical approach.

The new division would get an annual subsidy starting at $260,000 (the previous subsidy to contracted ambulance companies was $18,000 in 1970[4]), plus a one-time $200,000 capital injection for equipment and facilities to support six ambulances by day and three by night. The near future would reveal a rather more expensive service than originally projected.

To address demand for better medical care, the report urged the creation of a medical committee to determine medical training and qualifications for ambulance driver attendants and to train them to the level of an emergency medical technician. It also endorsed a

---

2 Park, Gary. "Ambulance Review Set." *Calgary Herald*, July 9, 1970. Accessed Aug. 14, 2018. https://news.google.com/newspapers?id=t-GxkAAAAIBAJ&sjid=CX0NAAAAI-BAJ&pg=1560,2497868.

3 "Citizens' Emergency Medical Services Advisory Committee Memo." Eric Musgreave, Tom Priddle, and Robt. Greene to His Worship Mayor Rod Sykes and Members of Council. November 12, 1970. In *Bill McComb Archive*.

4 Park. "Ambulance Review Set."

THE PRIVATE AMBULANCE ERA PRE-1971

City-appointed medical director to oversee the medical aspects of the service, including training, equipment and vehicle design.[5]

The owners of Aaron Ambulance pushed back against the City's initial offer to buy them out. They had struggled for years with bill collection and wanted enough to cover their losses. The City had publicly criticized the existing ambulance companies and Dr. Cohen bit back. Cohen and Richard Sigurdson negotiated with the City and finally agreed to sell, as long as they agreed to hire Sigurdson and have him help with the transition. While Cohen's visionary approach to ambulance care would have seemed to put him high on the list to be medical director for the new division, his clashes with the City had made him persona non grata. He moved his career to Montreal after the company's sale.

City council accepted the report, and effective Jan. 31, 1971, the City of Calgary's Ambulance Division opened for business.

---

5 Musgrave. "Citizens' Advisory Committee Memo."

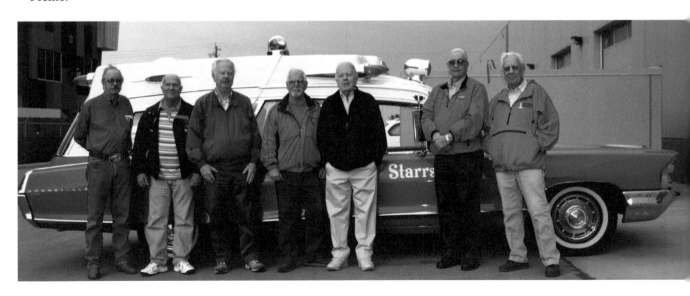

At an annual reunion of retired ambulance attendants and medics organized by Gary Fisher, these gentlemen were reunited with a piece of their past. They got to slide into the driver's seat of this Superior Pontiac, sister car to the ambulance most of them drove in the 1960s. From left: Sean Staddon, Gary Fisher, Bruce Castle, Randy Risdahl, Paddy Morrison, Fred Underhill, Clay Switzer. (Courtesy of Tim Prieur)

THE CALGARY FIRE DEPARTMENT ERA 1971-1984

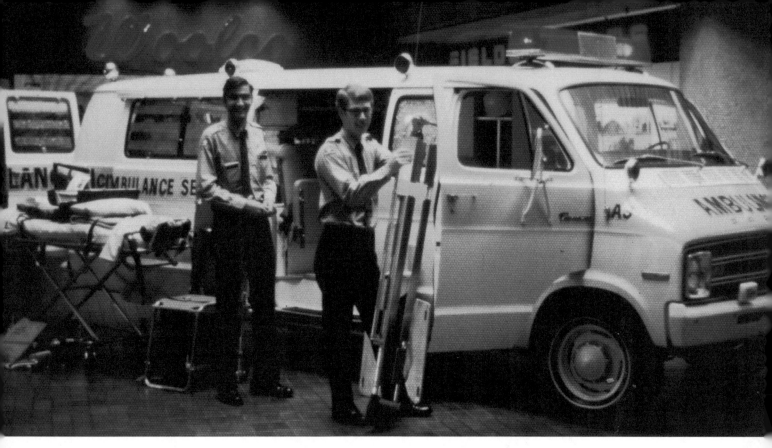

Two of Calgary's first paramedics, Rejean Denis (left) and Bill McComb set up for some citizen outreach in the mid-1970s. (Courtesy of Bill McComb)

THE CALGARY PARAMEDIC IS BORN

The birth of the City of Calgary Ambulance Division was the beginning of this city's world-class reputation for emergency medical services. But a lot of homework was required first. In taking over ambulance service, the City also raised the standard of training. Dr. Bill Donald was a pioneer in extracurricular education for those emergency vehicle operators who were interested in improving their skills, but buy-in for additional medical education wasn't exactly universal, at least not right away. Bill McComb was stationed in Fire Station #1 in downtown Calgary on one occasion when Donald stopped by to provide some training to the City employees. McComb—a few years away from becoming a paramedic—watched Donald demonstrate how to take a patient's blood pressure,

THE CALGARY FIRE DEPARTMENT ERA 1971–1984

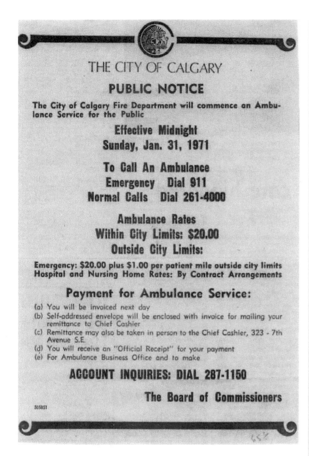

This notice appeared in print in 1971, signalling to the public a shift that they might only ever notice if and when they were to call an ambulance. (Courtesy of Tim Prieur)

thinking, "What the hell do we need to know this shit for?" Change was coming to the job, and it was coming fast.

By the spring of 1971, all Ambulance Division staff could take a pre-paramedical care course. It was a 60-hour program covering first aid, anatomy, physiology and some rescue techniques, instructed by fire department District Chief Bill Phillips and local doctors and firefighters. The top students would be able to attend a unique training program in Canada the following year, the Southern Alberta Institute of Technology's (SAIT) new Emergency Medical Technician Program. The SAIT program was in part a brainchild of Fire Chief Derek Jackson, who saw a lot of potential in his ambulance men. Jackson was well-liked by the newest members of the fire department. He cared about all the men in his employ, no matter if they were dousing fires or performing CPR. Firefighting is a brotherhood that doesn't easily welcome outsiders into their home. Jackson led the way in connecting the two groups. When a member of the fire department hockey team—a young ambulance man named Bob Willis—talked to Jackson about switching over to fire, Jackson told him he was too good at public relations between fire and ambulance. He convinced Willis to take the SAIT EMT course instead and serve as a connector between the two new neighbours.

The SAIT course initially consisted of six months in school and then later a three-month

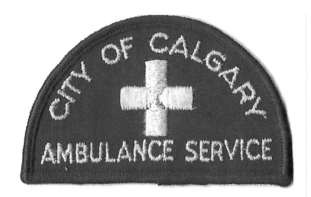

The first shoulder crest worn by the City of Calgary Ambulance Service, from 1971. (Courtesy of Bill McComb)

practicum. "The City went about it in the right way," said Gary Fisher. "We didn't worry about transporting bodies anymore. You weren't a bill collector anymore. You were taking care of people with more knowledge (than you'd ever had before)." The training also had the effect of keeping people in the profession longer than they had in the private ambulance days—they knew more, cared more and enjoyed it more.

The initial 22 EMT students had been ambulance drivers and attendants, had on-the-job experience and tended to be in their mid-to-late 20s. Today, most students apply straight out of high school with perhaps less overall life experience. At first, all students were employees of the Ambulance Division of the fire department, who worked while going to school. By the third intake class, members of the public were allowed to apply and attend.

The course was instructed by Janet Foster, RN. She told the *Calgary Herald* in 1972[6] the course was in part about learning the theory behind the practices they already used in their jobs. "They've already learned, through practical experience, how to perform certain emergency measures. Now they are learning why the measure is taken."

Dr. Bill Donald agreed the time had come for more training, telling the *Herald*: "Ambulance people deal with life and death all the time. They must be trained to handle any emergency until a doctor can take over. The patient should be delivered to the hospital certainly in no worse shape than the ambulance attendant found him."

The training was superior to anything offered to ambulance crews before. Richard Sigurdson, a graduate of the first class, said SAIT's training in anatomy, physiology and pharmacology was excellent. The one shortfall was that the working ambulance attendants knew far more about using a stretcher at the scene of a traumatic incident and other practical parts of their job than their instructors. Sigurdson's class built an ambulance out of plywood to use as a model. There were no preceptors available because

---

6 Whiteley, Don. "Ambulance Problems Over Now City's in the Driver's Seat." *Calgary Herald*, June 24, 1972. Accessed Aug 14, 2018. https://news.google.com/newspapers?id=nW9kAAAAI-BAJ&sjid=g30NAAAAIBAJ&pg=1230,1763718.

THE CALGARY FIRE DEPARTMENT ERA 1971–1984

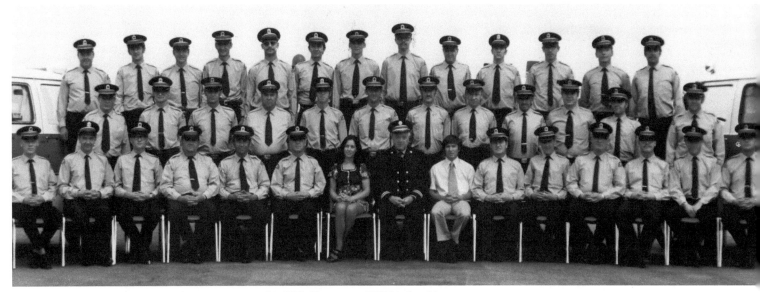

City of Calgary Ambulance Service personnel in 1971. (Courtesy of Bill McComb)

the training was just so new, so the students precepted one another. They learned how to start IVs at the Calgary General Hospital and did practicums in the emergency room (where many paramedics met their future wives who were nurses) and in obstetrics and psychology.

There were no protocols for these medics of the early 1970s. Protocols are essentially flowcharts of what to do in particular medical situations. Students in the SAIT program were taught what they could do and why, but were left to their own devices as to how to react in any given situation. Today, paramedics follow a thick book of 139 protocols guiding them in most emergencies. No protocols meant there was variation in the field from medic to medic; paramedics had to adapt to every emergency as it developed. In practice, you might get different treatment depending on which crew attended to you. Just as you might get different treatment between two physicians at the time.

The first SAIT Emergency Medical Technician Program students in 1972 attended school during the day and worked the city ambulances at night. By day, they studied all advanced life support materials available at time, including but not limited to IV solutions; medications and narcotics; intracardiac epinephrine injections (an injection straight into the heart's ventricles that you might recognize from the movie *Pulp Fiction*. The procedure was phased out due to the complications of possible damage to the heart.); ECG monitoring and interpretation; defibrillation; and endotracheal intubation. By night they were very sleepy.

To help each other catch at least a bit of sleep during this hectic school and work schedule, the staff used a rover car system. The rover car was a single ambulance responsible for every call overnight. The rover car crew started their shift at 1730, got some sleep until 2300 if they could, then covered calls across the city. They hovered around downtown for the best access to the rest of the city. As long as it didn't get too busy, it meant their fellow students could get some rest between work and school. Still, it wasn't unusual to find students asleep at their desks. It wasn't ideal, but it was the only way there were enough staffers to cover the city at the time. For later classes, the schedule was eased so students only had to work night shifts on the weekend, rather than pulling constant all-nighters, although the balance between school and work shifted through the years as the program evolved. From "ambulance drivers" and "emergency vehicle operators" a few months earlier, these students earned themselves new skills and a new title. Graduates were briefly known as Emergency Medical Technicians, or EMTs. But then the term "emergency paramedic," which was used only in the United States, was popularized internationally by the television show *Emergency!* It stuck. By 1973, SAIT changed the name of the program to the Paramedical Care Program and offered past graduates new certificates bearing the "Emergency Medical Technicians-Paramedic" title. The program was the first in Canada to graduate paramedics.

But in many ways, these paramedics graduated into a world where there was no space for them. "We're the new kids on the block, really," said Claude Belobersycky, an early graduate. "Nobody knew who we were. Nobody understood us, knew how to take us. Doctors looked at us funny… it was a real pioneering experience."

It would take years of effort for Calgary's paramedics to be understood by other first responders and the medical community. In hospitals, doctors often doubted their abilities while nurses were sometimes affronted that these former ambulance drivers were now doing procedures that even they were not allowed to do.

In fire halls, it wasn't unusual for some of their fire colleagues to see them as glorified first-aiders driving expensive ambulances. And the public, unless they had received care from one of these new paramedics, had next to no idea what they did. It was the beginning of a new era and there were trails to be blazed.

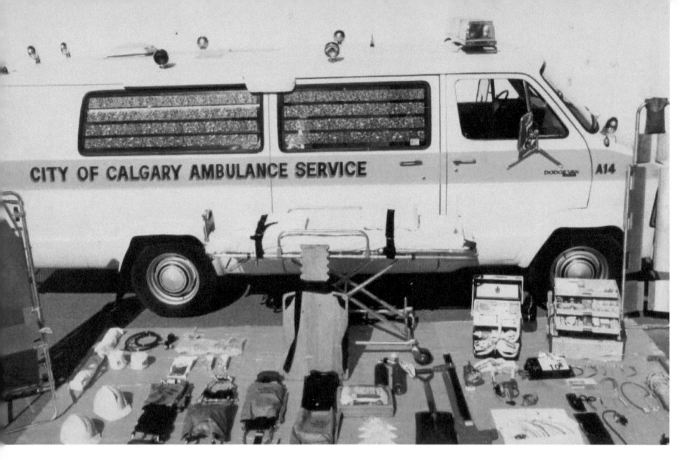

Along with new paramedic training came more and better equipment on ambulances in the mid-1970s. (Courtesy of Bill McComb)

"WHAT DO YOU NEED ALL THAT CRAP FOR?" NEXT-GENERATION AMBULANCE EQUIPMENT

Calgary's new paramedics had excellent training, but almost no advanced life support equipment on their ambulances and no drugs. In fact, for a while they had little more on their ambulance than they'd had in the private ambulance days. The City eventually purchased new gear and drugs to match their paramedics' training in 1973/74, but there was a hitch: provincial legislation didn't allow paramedics to perform the life-saving procedures they were educated to carry out. "It was unquestionably frustrating," said Ron McManus. The government didn't get around to updating the relevant legislation until 1986.

THE CALGARY FIRE DEPARTMENT ERA 1971–1984

Until the new laws were enacted, a workaround was required to allow paramedics to provide life-saving treatment at the scene. Beginning in 1974, paramedics were permitted to do several advanced life-saving procedures—but only if they had medical control or a "patch," meaning they were in radio or phone contact with an emergency room physician. With a patch, they could perform cardiac monitoring and defibrillation, administer IVs and parenteral injections of drugs (meaning drugs that weren't taken orally, including injections into the heart), endotracheal intubation (maintaining an open trachea by inserting a flexible tube down the windpipe) and intermittent positive pressure breathing (for a patient who is not breathing properly). Without patching, they could take a patient's blood pressure.

Needing a doctor's oversight wasn't unique to the ambulance service. Doctors have long been at the top of the medical hierarchy and it's only recently that they've relinquished certain duties to nurses, paramedics and other specialists. While technically paramedics weren't allowed to do any type of advanced life support without being on the line with the doctor, in practice, more-experienced paramedics were known to go ahead and do their best to save lives before picking up the phone. You couldn't always wait around when someone's heart had stopped. In the earliest days of medical control, the radio system could only handle talking in one direction at a time.

The paramedic might have to repeat their request—"General Hospital, this is Paramedic 1, over"—several times before a doctor could answer if he was busy suturing. Often, an RN would answer the call and it wasn't unusual for there to be issues with the modem, meaning an ECG couldn't be printed or given to a doctor to read. It was a frustrating process, to say the least. Ideally, the paramedic would radio EMS dispatch, who would phone the hospital to advise that the paramedic wanted a voice patch on phone or radio, then a nurse or unit clerk would track down the appropriate doctor. When a paramedic was able to speak directly to a doctor, the doctor's instructions might be incredibly basic, like, "Open the airway and start CPR." (A gratingly obvious action.) On the other hand, a different doctor might ask if an IV had been started and what did the ECG look like—except the paramedic wasn't supposed to start an IV without the doctor's oversight. It was far from consistent and a paramedic never knew whom they would get on the line.

Many doctors didn't yet trust paramedics' abilities. Ron McManus recalled a particular doctor whose only response to a call from a paramedic was, "Bring him in!" McManus got that exact response while responding to a call for chest pain 90 minutes outside the city. He believed his patient needed treatment immediately, not after a 90-minute drive to the hospital. So McManus called his dispatcher and asked to talk to a doctor at the General Hospital instead. "This isn't exactly following the rules,"

VITAL SIGNS

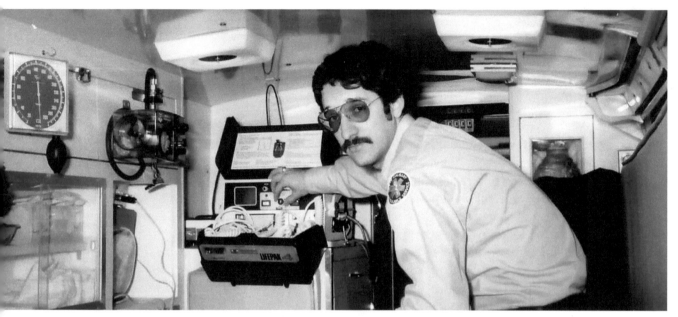

Paramedic Gary Marlatt works inside a City of Calgary ambulance unit alongside essential gear, including a Lifepak 4 monitor/defibrillator and a Bird Mark 7 Respirator. (Courtesy of Bill McComb)

said McManus. "But there weren't any rules." "Shopping for doctor's orders" became the standard of practice by the mid-1970s.

Ambulances were filling up with more gear and gadgets to complement paramedics' skills. There would, as ever, be a regular stretcher and auxiliary stretcher onboard. The latter could be attached to the bench seat in the back of the ambulance in case it needed to carry a second patient. A spine board and a short spine board were standard, too. Typically, they were made of three-quarter-inch varnished plywood with holes cut out for straps to be attached, to secure a patient with a suspected neck or spine injury. Military Anti-Shock Trousers (MAST pants) were also onboard. Before the fire department could cut roofs off vehicles, the short spine board was used when paramedics needed to extricate patients.

New to the ambulances were advanced Lifepak 4 heart monitors and defibrillators. These devices were hefty, weighing around 30 pounds. The most advanced part of the Lifepak 4 was the modem, which allowed paramedics to transmit ECG signals to a hospital for a doctor to read and provide instructions remotely.

THE CALGARY FIRE DEPARTMENT ERA 1971–1984

The paramedic first aid kit had grown from the basic black leather doctor's bag of gauze, bandages and airways to enough supplies to fit in a large fishing tackle box. Eventually, the company making the tackle boxes customized a version specifically for medical use, called the Plano 747. The big white and orange plastic case was always full of supplies and as a bonus, it doubled as an extra seat (albeit not a particularly safe one) for a practicum student.

Taking blood pressure was now standard, so the Plano 747 contained a blood pressure cuff and stethoscope. It held an intubation kit with a laryngoscope, various sizes of blades and plastic tubing. For years, the reusable intubation kit was contained in a custom cloth roll until eventually sterile packaging and single-use scopes came around.

All the paraphernalia required for IVs, including needles, tubes and solutions were in the tackle box. The bag valve resuscitator, which was a mask with a bag attached that could be squeezed to force air into a patient's lungs, was brand-new to ambulance work.

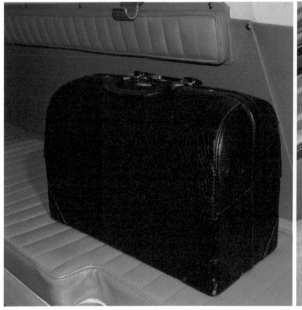 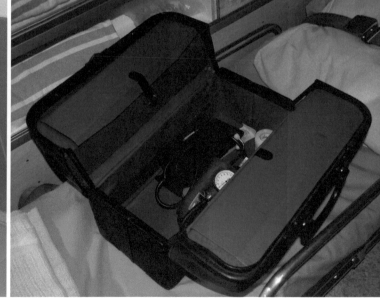

A medical bag stocked on ambulances in 1972. (Courtesy of Tim Prieur)

Eventually, oxygen could be attached to it for use when resuscitating a patient.

Calgary ambulances for the first time began carrying drugs. "It was slow getting started," said Bill McComb. "Before we got the drugs, we had the training (to use them) and we sure wished we had morphine we could give." McComb once attended to a call at a restaurant where a man using a meat grinder got his hand caught in the machine. He was in excruciating pain. The best they could offer the man was to transport him—the meat grinder still attached—to the hospital. There, doctors were finally able to administer morphine and, with the assistance of the fire department rescue team, turn the grinder in reverse to free his hand. In time, ambulances carried morphine and Demerol for pain control, along with a variety of what one paramedic called "speeder-uppers and slower-downers;" in other words, cardiac drugs. The speeder-uppers included atropine and intra-cardiac epinephrine. Atropine was also used to treat organophosphate exposure, for example certain weed-killing agents. Paramedics used intravenous sodium bicarbonate "by the bucketful" said McComb, for when the heart stopped and the body became acidotic, but it later fell out of usage. Lidocaine was used mostly intravenously to treat ventricular fibrillation (cardiac arrest), but could also be used in aerosol form as a local anesthetic in the throat when intubating. Isoproterenol was used to treat cardiac conditions and, less often, asthma patients. Other drugs on the ambulance would have included anti-convulsants, more cardiac meds and anti-histamines. They also carried several types of IV solutions: normal saline, D5W, D5W with Lidocaine and Ringer's Lactate.

Overall, between vastly improved training and equipment, the impact on care was dramatic and Calgary's paramedic service was being noticed around the country. That notice wasn't always roundly positive. Initially, nurses in Calgary were a bit disgruntled about these upstart paramedics suddenly being able to provide ALS care that even they weren't doing at that point, such as administering drugs intravenously or intubating patients. Whether it was jealousy or mistrust, it soon faded as the nursing community began to see the impact on patients and the ability to work as part of a team with the paramedics.

Calgary's service was a microcosm of advanced care in the early 1970s. While the city's paramedics trailblazed, the private ambulance crews in Edmonton scoffed. Up north, they were still a scoop and run service operating out of customized Cadillac and Oldsmobile ambulances administering "glorified first aid." "They were back in the dark ages in Edmonton," said Ron McManus. After transferring a patient to Edmonton once, McManus and his partner came back to their ambulance to see a couple of their Edmonton counterparts scoping out all the gear: the

THE CALGARY FIRE DEPARTMENT ERA 1971–1984

Bird Mark 7 Respirator mask, the defibrillator, cabinets full of drugs. One of the fellows turned to the Calgary crew and said, "What do you need all that crap for?" The attitude was that if their car could go 130 km/h, they could get to the hospital before their patient died.

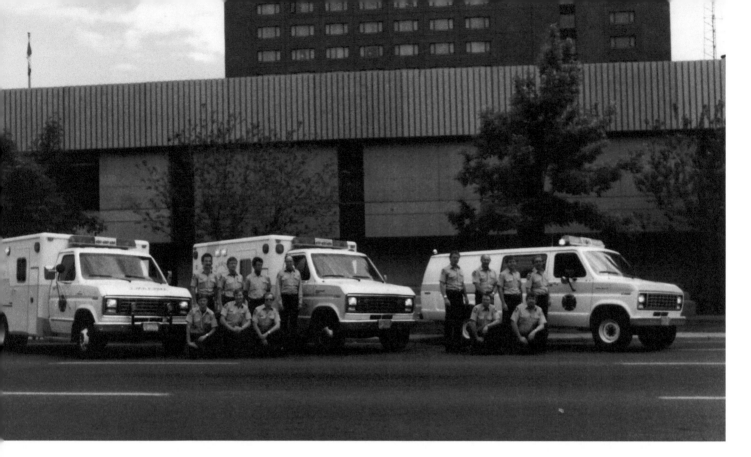

Modular ambulances, such as the two units at left, were nice and roomy. Platoon members appreciated the extra storage and space to work on patients. They were considered by most members to be a step above van units. (Courtesy of Bill McComb)

VANS, MODS AND THE BEAST

There was some experimentation required when it came to finding the ideal ambulance vehicle for the new service. The old custom ambulances were not big enough. The City's first ambulances were low-roof Ford vans. They were painted with a red stripe and gold lettering to match the fire department. The department later switched to Dodge vans that were longer and faster, but still had a low roof. "Our superintendent didn't see the need for a high roof when you were always sitting down anyway," said Bill McComb. "Besides, you could brace your shoulders on the ceiling while you did CPR." These ambulances were painted with a lime yellow stripe to co-ordinate with the fire department's new colour scheme.

THE CALGARY FIRE DEPARTMENT ERA 1971–1984

Paramedic Gary Fisher set the ambulance service's one official land speed record in one of those Dodge vans. Fisher was responding from Station #17, north of the University of Calgary, headed to Morley, AB. RCMP clocked him at 188 km/h. He retrieved his patient and on his way to Foothills hospital, he was again clocked at the same speed by the same officers, who had moved their radar to the other side of the highway. (This was accomplished within the hour as per land speed record criteria.)

The RCMP officers were so impressed they packed up the radar and followed the ambulance to the hospital to congratulate Fisher. It's worth noting that current policy stipulates that an ambulance must not exceed the posted speed limit by more than 15 km/h.

In most ambulance models, stretchers were mounted on the left side of the vehicle, so paramedics could only access one side of the patient from the squad bench. The bench performed a triple function: it could seat two

This unit, A1, was the first new ambulance ordered by the City of Calgary to build its fleet in 1971. (Courtesy of Bill McComb)

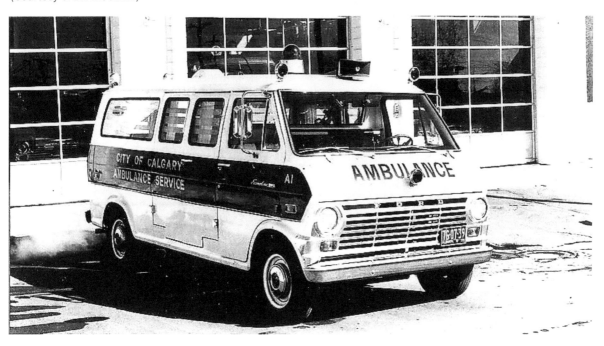

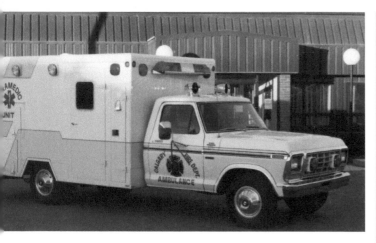

A13, also known as "The Beast," was an early modular ambulance used by the City. The "box" on the back was the most expensive part of the unit, so theoretically, the ambulance could be driven for a few years, and then the box swapped onto a new chassis. (Courtesy of Bill McComb)

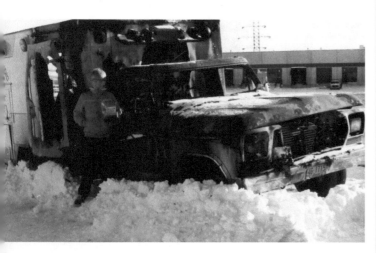

But unit A13 did not get a new lease on life. It was thoroughly burned on the side of a highway. (Courtesy of Bill McComb)

or three people, had brackets to fit a portable stretcher in case a second patient needed transport, and held storage underneath.

The staff wanted bigger vehicles to facilitate the emergency medical services they provided. The amount of equipment and supplies they carried had at least doubled in the decade since the City took over. By 1979, the department purchased six modular ambulance models (known as "mods") from six different suppliers to test. Most of them were "boxes" mounted on a van chassis, much like what you see on Calgary streets today. One of the six trial units was built on a truck chassis and earned the nickname "The Beast" because it was so cumbersome and heavy. Almost nobody liked The Beast. On one bitterly cold winter day, a paramedic crew was transferring a patient on Highway 2 when the truck caught fire. As the cab started to fill with smoke, paramedic John Amat pulled over and helped his partner get the patient out of the back of the unit in a blustery -20 C. A snowplow truck stopped to help and provide them shelter until the local fire department could come extinguish the fire. "Paramedic Amat was hailed as a hero," wrote Bill McComb. "Not just for helping rescue the patient, but mostly for ensuring that The Beast went up in flames."

Other than The Beast, the spacious modular ambulances were a hit with the staff and great for morale.

VITAL SIGNS

A DAY IN THE LIFE OF CALGARY'S FIRST PARAMEDICS

In 1971, the Calgary Fire Department's Ambulance Division had five ambulances covering a city of 400,000 people during the day and three on overnight. The paramedics were spread a little thin and kept on their toes, but they weren't nearly as busy as Calgary's paramedics today. They operated out of three fire stations: #1 in downtown Calgary, #16 in the Highfield industrial area and #7 on 4th Street and 26th Avenue N.W.. The 1970s saw a population explosion in Calgary, fuelled by rocketing oil prices, with a 45% increase in population from 1970 to 1980—and call volumes rose, too. By 1974, there were six fire stations housing the ambulance service, growing to 21 by the 1980s.

A typical day shift included chores at the fire station from 0900–1000 hours. The routine varied, though chores would typically include both crew members cleaning the car and the hall. Nine times out of 10, the ambulance would receive a call around chores o'clock, which rubbed some firefighters the wrong way.

When they handed over their patients to the emergency room, paramedics would also pass along a patient care report, or PCR. This was an advancement in record-keeping compared to the past, but much of what was recorded could be easily shared with the nurse face to face and the PCR was often stuffed at the back of the patient's medical chart, never to be seen again. (Courtesy of Bill McComb)

THE CALGARY FIRE DEPARTMENT ERA 1971–1984

Whether it was a real call or an excuse to miss chores may have varied. It was, after all, a busy city out there.

The Ambulance Division uniform included a light blue shirt with a red shoulder crest reading "City of Calgary Ambulance Service," a black tie and a short-brimmed black hat. The hat was widely regarded as completely impractical and was roundly despised and ignored by most ambulance staffers. It resembled a police officer's hat, but with a red and white stripe around it. In fact, the resemblance to a police officer was an issue; certain patients definitely didn't want to see a police officer approaching them and a situation might escalate if they thought one was. In fact, while the hats were part of the uniform, they were so rarely worn that they once helped solve an ambulance theft. A crew was tending to a patient and returned to the spot where they'd parked their ambulance to find it missing. The culprit was later tracked down—identified in part because he'd found a hat in the ambulance and put it on his head as a disguise. In another case, a crew responded to a motor vehicle collision outside the city on a windy day. A hat-hating medic on the call tossed his hat away and let the wind blow it into a farmer's field. He happily went about his work for a couple days until the farmer found it and returned it to the fire department.

The necktie was a whole other issue. It was susceptible to dangling in a patient's face while a paramedic was trying to work. But worse, it

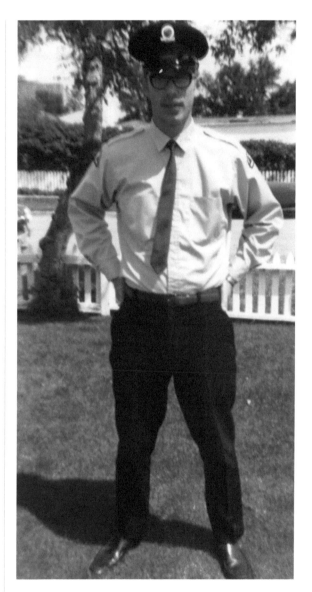

In 1971, a paramedic's tie and hat were likely to be the least-loved pieces of his uniform.
(Courtesy of Bill McComb)

43

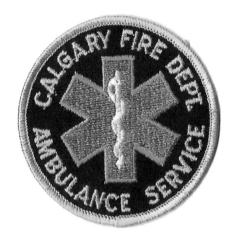

It was hoped that a redesigned shoulder patch would help strengthen ties between the fire department and ambulance service. The yellow stitching around the edge of this patch denotes it was worn by a supervisor. (Courtesy of Tim Prieur)

was a serious choking hazard when dealing with a distressed or psychotic patient. "They could kill you with that tie," said McManus. Eventually the tie was switched to a safer clip-on version.

The patch on the uniform shirt evolved over the years. There was a round black patch with a complementary rocker designating whether the wearer was an EMT or a paramedic. Later, in an attempt to make the Ambulance Division feel more a part of the fire department, the patch was changed to say "Calgary Fire Department Ambulance Service." This did little to build the relationship between the two groups.

Depending who you ask, you might hear that Calgarians in the '70s tended to look after their own problems more than they do now. The ambulances covering downtown were regularly called to alcohol-related emergencies, assaults and drug overdoses. Heroin was a particular problem throughout the '70s, reaching epidemic levels for about 18 months starting in 1973. Bill McComb recalled being anxious heading to his first heroin overdose call. A particularly potent supply had hit the streets. McComb was working with a new recruit who was anxious to attend to his first heroin call. McComb wanted to put his partner at ease and took a guess at what they could expect. "Not to worry," he said. "Their breathing will get slower and slower and then they'll stop. Then we use a bag valve mask on them to help them breathe and then they'll wake up and be mad at us for waking them up from this great dream they were having." McComb predicted it exactly right. By 1975, ambulances were carrying the anti-overdose drug Narcan (naloxone). Heroin wasn't the only drug concern. Valium, Librium and other tranquilizers were popular prescriptions at the time that led to abuse and accidental overdoses.

A shift might include eight to 15 calls, considerably more than decades later thanks to quick drop-offs at the hospital. Typically, it was a quick transition from ambulance stretcher to hospital bed. The paramedics would have a brief conversation with the nurse to relay treatment to that point and then be back on the road. While paramedics of the day had many more skills and equipment than they had a decade earlier, plenty of what they did was still transporting patients to hospital. At least, if the patient wanted to go, that is. A patient could refuse transport to hospital and some paramedics would essentially shrug and appreciate having less paperwork. It would be a few more years before a patient had to sign a waiver if they refused treatment or transport.

When it was particularly busy, the fire department would be dispatched to provide basic life support (BLS) until an ambulance could attend. This type of situation highlighted an ongoing issue for the Ambulance Division: who was in charge at the scene of a medical emergency? Was it the fire captain—who had seniority at the fire hall—or the paramedic with the extensive medical training and experience? Ron McManus recalled one incident where this clash was particularly concerning. McManus and his partner arrived on the scene of a cardiac incident where the fire department was providing basic life support. McManus intended to follow the typical procedure, by bringing oxygen, defibrillator, ECG and first aid kit into the home upon arrival—but a firefighter standing outside the home shouted at them to bring in a stretcher. McManus ignored the insistent firefighter. Inside, one firefighter was performing chest compressions while the other was blowing air on his mouth—in other words, they were not properly ventilating the patient and McManus told them so. The fire captain at the scene insisted the current actions were correct and became livid when the paramedics ignored his orders. Eventually, the paramedics determined it was time to transport the patient to the hospital. They moved him onto the stretcher and into the ambulance.

As McManus was about to drive away with his patient, the fire captain told him to take the patient to the Colonel Belcher Hospital. McManus had already spoken to a doctor at the General and that's where he was going; he told the captain as much. (The Belcher, a veterans' hospital, didn't have an emergency department, nor was it staffed by physicians 24/7.) As McManus pulled away, he heard a thunk—the fire captain was hammering on the back of the ambulance. In a meeting with the district chief after the fact, McManus was able to convince the higher-up his medical opinion was the one that mattered in the scenario. The district chief agreed, telling the captain, "You're supposed to support the paramedic, not fight them." But it didn't make a difference with that guy going forward.

"AMBULANCE PROBLEMS OVER"

In June 1972, the *Calgary Herald*[7] published an article with the bold headline, "Ambulance Problems Over now City's in the Driver's Seat." As you might guess, it was a bombastic statement. Just try to find an ambulance service anywhere in the world without headaches. But compared to the Universal Ambulance strike of 1970 or the fights over patients, the service was exceptional. The article noted that the $400,000 annual cost to the city (in 1972 dollars) was much more than the previous $15,000 subsidy they provided in their contract for private ambulance service—but it was worth every penny according to Division Chief Bill Phillips. Their gear was better, their training vastly improved, paramedics were able to prioritize patient care and transport rather than play bill collector, and they had benefits. The division had nine vehicles, 52 attendants/paramedics and three stations. But the service still had lofty goals ahead, including creating a uniform fleet of ambulance vehicles and upgrading their resuscitation equipment.

While the members of the Ambulance Division were busy with the professionalization of their careers, there was some chafing happening back at the fire halls through the 1970s. The at times casual, laid-back men who were hired from the ambulance companies were not always a perfect fit in the quasi-military context of the fire department. It was a complicated relationship, probably made worse by the inadvertent class divide the City had made when it created the division within the fire department. Ambulance personnel were "fire civilians." "We always felt like we were second-class citizens," said Bill McComb. McComb said there was a different mindset between the fire and ambulance groups: "A paramedic was trained to be an individual thinker. They just go off and do their own thing all the time. 'They have no discipline,' a firefighter might say. A firefighter is trained to be part of a group, follow orders and work together as part of a crew. That's how they survive in the fire and in the station."

As education qualifications increased for paramedics, there wasn't a commensurate pay increase. Paramedics with the same years of experience were making less than the firefighters, despite more training. Gino Savoia had enrolled at SAIT in 1978, inspired to try emergency medicine as a career after catching an episode of the popular TV show *Emergency!*

---

7 Whiteley. "Ambulance Problems Over."

THE CALGARY FIRE DEPARTMENT ERA 1971–1984

It looked exciting and his tuition would be paid for by the City. He didn't realize he'd have to work a second job during school to pay the bills. He hadn't always thought EMTs were cool. In fact, Savoia was attending SAIT studying film & TV when the EMT program launched. He and his fellow self-described "longhairs" thought the ambulance guys, who wore white smock uniforms with a pill collar and plastic pocket protectors and could be seen practicing putting stretchers into a wooden ambulance, were serious nerds. But years later, he was ready to join the club.

He wrote a pre-employment general aptitude test for the fire department along with just 11 other people (today similar tests run by the City for firefighters get thousands of applicants). By that point, the SAIT program had expanded into two years and 2,700+ hours. Savoia worked at a pizzeria during school while also working for the City. He made less than $3.50 an hour working for the City, but $6.50 hourly at the pizza place. "You can see how skewed the pay grid was," said Savoia. Firefighters were making $5.70 an hour at the same time.

VITAL SIGNS

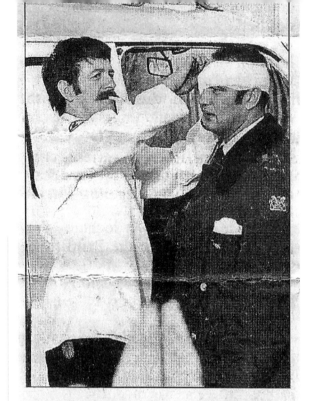

An emergency worker attends to an officer with a head wound.

Paramedic Bob Willis was just trying to get through a terrifying day at work when a newspaper photographer snapped this moment of relative calm during a storm of bullets. (Courtesy of Postmedia News/Bill McComb)

BLACK FRIDAY

Paramedics had long had a positive relationship with the Calgary Police Service, but one tragic day cemented those ties. On Dec. 20, 1974, police responded to a call from a shopkeeper who, after selling multiple tubes of model airplane glue to a man over the previous week, had declined to him sell any more. The man turned abusive and the shopkeeper phoned the police.

When the police arrived, they learned the man was wanted on a warrant, but he refused to get into their car. Instead, Phillipe Gagnon, who was visibly deranged after sniffing glue for days, returned to the garage of his home. Three officers entered the garage, intending to apprehend him. But constables Harvey Gregorash, Mel Lynn and Tom Dick didn't know Gagnon had a cache of modified guns. They also didn't know he was hunkered down in a recess in the floor, probably originally designed for doing mechanical work. When the officers entered the garage, Gagnon aimed a shot at them. His gun misfired, but in the subsequent moments, Gagnon shot two of the officers. One bullet struck Dick right where his wallet was—his billfold saving him from worse injury.[8] The other hit Gregorash in the head. Lynn and Dick escaped, then went back to pull Gregorash to safety. They were under fire and returning fire. That's about when paramedics received a rare call: police officer shot.

---

8 Smith, Peter. "Heroes Were Born in the City's Deadliest Shootout 25 Years Ago." *Calgary Sun*, Dec. 19, 1999.

THE CALGARY FIRE DEPARTMENT ERA 1971–1984

"I don't remember being afraid at the scene," said Richard Sigurdson, who was a superintendent for the Ambulance Division at the time. "We had absolutely no plan. There was no plan for that kind of an incident. My plan was the seat of my pants."

When paramedic Bob Willis and his partner Doug Davis arrived, the scene was already mass chaos. "Police started showing up from everywhere and the war was on," Willis said. Bullets and tear gas canisters filled the air. Willis had just completed his paramedic training at SAIT months earlier. He knew he was part of a group of pioneering medics, but he never expected to be in the midst of a shootout in Calgary. Willis said there was no time to be terrified. "You were busy, so you didn't have that much time," he said. "I know what the sound of a bullet is going by your ear." Willis was photographed by a newspaper photographer, a cigarette hanging out of his mouth as he re-affixed the bandage around Gregorash's head. Technically, he wasn't supposed to be smoking while working with a patient. Willis said his thought in that moment was, "I'll quit smoking when he quits shooting."

Police weapons were unable to penetrate the shooter's makeshift bunker in the garage. Nothing like this had ever happened in Calgary and the police didn't have the tactical equipment or strategies to respond. Gagnon used modified guns with automatic shooting capability, firing high-velocity rounds. They ripped through the garage and through police cruisers. His shots wounded officers Bob Barrett, Kip Sylvester and Nick Graham. Det. Boyd Davidson was shot in the head, a wound that proved to be fatal. Davidson was the first Calgary Police member killed in the line of duty in 40 years.

The tear gas, it was later found, had no effect on Gagnon due to the detrimental effects of glue sniffing on his airways and tear ducts. Meanwhile, it was burning the eyes of police and paramedics.

Officer Nick Graham was shot in the head, and had to be helped to a nearby ambulance while bullets flew. Despite the protests of the ambulance attendants, he walked himself from the vehicle into the emergency department where his friend, a neurosurgeon, later chided him for getting so much dirt in his head wound.[9]

Over the course of the day, 130 police officers were involved, 60 were directly in the line of fire, shooting nearly 1,000 bullets and hurling 67 tear gas canisters into Gagnon's house and garage.[10] Eight officers were shot. Det. Boyd Davidson was the sole officer killed.

---

9 " 'Please Don't Die on Me'." *Calgary Sun*, Dec. 19, 1999.

10 D'Amour, Peter. "Black Friday." *Calgary Sun*, Dec. 19, 2004.

"There were gunshots while we were trying to get Boyd Davidson out of there," said Sigurdson. "They were shooting right around us and over our heads. It wasn't until it was over and I was driving home, scared shitless because then we knew what had happened."

"The evacuation process… that was dead-ass wrong… it's a wonder we never lost any (medics)," said Sigurdson. Calgary was plunged into the modern crime world that day. Police weapons couldn't pierce the garage door and finally, a call was made to Ottawa requesting military intervention. The army reserves arrived from Currie Barracks, crushing Gagnon's garage under the force of their armoured personnel carrier and forcing him out of his bunker. Gagnon was shot dead as he tried to escape.

"He had about 18 holes in him by the time we put him in an ambulance," said Sigurdson. Willis and Davis transferred Gagnon's body to the morgue, the day "all kind of a blur," Willis said.

The incident changed policing in Calgary, including spawning the creation of the force's tactical team starting the very next morning, when Police Chief Brian Sawyer sent men to Los Angeles to train with the SWAT team there. Decades later, it would also influence the creation of a Tactical EMS (TEMS) team. Willis said there were no psychological supports for the medics on the scene that day. "It wasn't a very good day," he said. But he did say there was a "1,000%" change between police and medics. They'd just been "ambulance guys" to the police before; now they were best buddies.

The fire halls were buzzing the next day. Everyone was asking the medics who'd been there what it had been like to be at the scene. Willis said he and the others who were there really didn't want to talk about it. "It wasn't a happy time," he said. Willis' contribution on Black Friday earned him the nickname "Bullet" the following morning. It immediately stuck. In fact, it stuck so well that he was allowed to update his name badge to read "Bullet."

The Ambulance Division did make some changes to their approach to active police situations. In the past, as on Dec. 20, 1974, medics rushed right into the heat of the action. New rules meant waiting in a safe zone, even if that meant leaving a patient waiting in distress for longer, "which is pretty hard," Bullet said.

Forty years later, Bullet and Davis were presented with the Police Chief's award for their exemplary service on Black Friday. They were the first civilians to receive the award.

AMBULANCE WOMEN

The job of an "ambulance man" was tough work. Not just because of the high-pressure, high-stakes medical circumstances, but also the patriarchy. In 1969, a Calgary editorial quoted Universal Ambulance manager John Morrison explaining many aspects of the job. He also touched on the lack of ambulance women.

"We've had women apply. But we don't accept them," he told the journalist. "Not because they couldn't qualify from a first aid point of view, but because it's a back-breaking job, literally. We have to carry 90 percent of our patients. Some of them are heavy. It's too much for a woman. Most ambulance attendants have injured their backs at one time or another.

"Then women would run into the old problem of the male ego. If an injured man saw a woman coming to carry him, he'd probably insist he could walk. He wouldn't want to be helped by a woman. It's silly, but that's the way people are." [11]

And that's the way people stayed, apparently, at least for a couple more years. A newspaper ad placed by the City of Calgary described their ideal candidate as follows: "Young men of good character and repute are invited to apply. Desired age 21 to 29 years inclusive, preferred height and weight 5'8" to 6'2", 160 lbs. to 190 lbs in balanced proportion. Absolute education minimum Grade 10." [12] The deadline to reply to the ad was Feb. 12, 1971.

By the late 1970s, Carolyn Kremer was completely set on becoming a paramedic. She'd started by taking a few nighttime first-aid courses from her ski club, but was so absorbed in the course material and stories from the paramedic who taught it, that she wanted to do more. Kremer signed up for an extended two-week EMT course provided by an American company in Banff and her fate was sealed. She didn't just want to learn all this stuff, she wanted to use it to help people.

Kremer had no sense of what that ad and editorial had said years earlier, and applied to the City. She'd just missed a batch of hiring and she was directed instead to apply to a computer-based EMT-A training program.

---

[11] (Calgary). "Ambulance Men Well Trained." Editorial. 1969.

[12] City of Calgary. "Ambulance Attendants (Trainees)." Advertisement. (Calgary), 1970/1.

THE CALGARY FIRE DEPARTMENT ERA 1971–1984

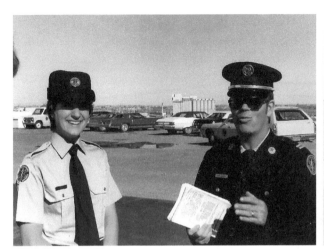
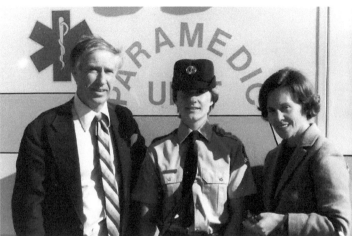

Carolyn Kremer, at left with Dave Jensen, and at right with her parents, was inspired to become a paramedic. In 1980, she became one of the first women hired into the City of Calgary Ambulance Division. (Courtesy of Bill McComb)

The remote program was developed by the Alberta Department of Advanced Education to extend a higher level of training to more Alberta ambulance services. It was shorter than the SAIT program, teaching basic life support (rather than advanced) and relying on self-guided learning using computers. Eventually, a practicum component on ambulances was added too. The following September, in 1980, she was hired as an EMT and became one of the first women to work in the Ambulance Division of the fire department. She didn't know it at the time, but Kremer had just begun her 32-year career in the ambulance service.

It was a "very macho culture," in the fire department at that time, Kremer said. But she didn't let that deter her from getting the job done. "I'm a very non-confrontational kind of person and I'm goal- and task-oriented. I was there to serve on the ambulance and that was my focus."

Bob "Bullet" Willis thought it was just fine having women around the fire department. After all, medics had been working alongside nurses who were women in Calgary for decades. He called them "pioneers, those women that first started. They could take it—and hand it out." Willis said that Fire Chief Jack Ross credited women paramedics for opening doors for women firefighters in Calgary.

Early on, Kremer clashed with one particular fire captain who already didn't like having the ambulance people around and certainly wasn't used to having a woman in the fire hall. He would complain about how she'd parked her ambulance and other digs like that. But then he started to notice that she was always on top of the chores around the fire hall that other paramedics and EMTs seemed to shirk and he started to come around. One day, he told her he'd spoken to her supervisor and asked that she always be assigned to his station. Later, he learned that they lived in the same neighbourhood and offered to carpool. It was proof that the two disparate groups could find their similarities. "It was just being yourself and not trying to change history," Kremer said. "And you could just kind of worm your way in and soon become part of the crew."

Different platoons had separate lockers in the firehall kitchen and a rather popular decoration were "sunshine girl" photos. Kremer, wanting to contribute to the decor, posted a complementary "sunshine boy". Her colleagues found it hilarious.

Women joining the ranks didn't always go smoothly. Kremer said she recalled some of her female colleagues through the years struggling with how to deal with inappropriate conduct at work. There weren't systems in place to address the issues and fighting it became futile. "You're fighting a big machine," she said. "They could make your life hell and you might not want to go that path." Kremer said that there was no protocol in place for parental leave; the first woman in the department to become pregnant quit and then was rehired after her baby was born. Later, pregnant medics stopped working on the ambulance at 20 weeks. Eventually, light duty was provided during the latter weeks.

Kremer had been working for the City as an EMT for two years by the time she'd earned the seniority required to head to SAIT for paramedic training. The balance between work and school was often in flux over the first decade of the program, and the start of Kremer's time was no exception. For at least a couple years, paramedic students did not have to work ambulance shifts while in school. Kremer and her classmates were informed that due to budgetary restrictions, they would be expected to work when not in class and get someone to cover their shift while they were in class. Kremer said there were times when she would pack her car with clothes to last her a whole week, she was so busy. "That year, my Christmas tree didn't come down 'til March and I had to dust the baubles to put them away," she said.

While Kremer and her classmates studied, trouble was brewing in the fire department.

THE CALGARY FIRE DEPARTMENT ERA 1971–1984

THE CITY OF CALGARY
requires
AMBULANCE ATTENDANTS (TRAINEES)
Fire Department
Ambulance Division
Competition No. 71-009

To establish an eligibility list to fill a number of permanent vacancies as they arise.

DUTIES:
Candidates who are accepted and placed on the eligibility list will be absorbed, on an as required basis, into the ambulance service as trainees. As a member of a team will be required, on a rotating shift basis, to drive and operate an ambulance in response to emergency or other service calls. To pick up sick, injured and convalescents and transport them to required destination. To perform related tasks as required or assigned. Hours of work will average 42 hours per week.

SALARY:
$430 (Trainee) - 460 - 490 - 520 - 550 - 580 - 610 per month.
Hours of work — average 42 hours per week on a rotating shift basis.

QUALIFICATIONS:
Young men of good character and repute are invited to apply. Desired age 21 to 29 years inclusive, preferred height and weight 5'8'' to 6'2'', 160 lbs. to 190 lbs. in balanced proportion. Absolute education minimum Grade X. Possession of valid "D" licence, Province of Alberta, with no restrictions as to ability to acquire an "A" licence. A sincere desire and proven interest in First Aid work, with a willingness to undertake additional practical and academic training in order to improve and standardize ambulance attendant qualifications. Please be prepared to present Alberta driver's licence and and First Aid achievement certificates on request.

APPLY:
Application forms are to be obtained from, and returned not later than 5:00 p.m. Friday, February 12, 1971, to:

Personnel Co-ordinator
The City of Calgary
P.O. Box 2100
Calgary 2, Alberta

503737

The City of Calgary sought "young men of good character and repute" to apply to be ambulance attendant trainees in 1971. A particular physique and a valid driver's licence were top requirements. (Courtesy of Tim Prieur)

THE PARAMEDIC WARS OF 1982

On Nov. 11, 1981, all the annoyances and concerns between fire and ambulance came to a head. About three months earlier, the Fire department had installed a new radio system designed specifically for the way they responded to fire calls. Previously, the Department—including ambulances—had been using a three-channel citywide radio system based on the Calgary Transit radio model. It was a bit noisy and coverage on the outskirts of town was spotty, but it worked well enough.

But the new system, while great for the way firefighters worked, just didn't suit the reality of emergency ambulance service. While fire crews worked out of a single station and returned to that station after a call, and therefore could use the same radio channel all shift, the opposite was true for paramedics. In practice, it meant it was a struggle for ambulance crews to communicate in the ways they needed to. Finally, on that Remembrance Day, a paramedic was frustrated enough with trying to use the radio that he instead used a payphone to patch to the hospital. The union found out and was livid that this radio system was affecting patients now, and complained to the City's chief commissioner, George Cornish.

Despite the holiday, Cornish acted immediately. He directed the fire department to immediately replace the ambulance radios with the previous system and it happened that very day.

For the ambulance service, the radio failure was a symbol of their perceived second-class status within the fire department. All their fears—that their functions were undervalued and misunderstood by fire captains, and that budget would be spent on re-upholstering a fire truck before it was spent on medical equipment—seemed to be confirmed. (The medical control board had recommended the ambulance service upgrade to new heart monitors that could print out more legible ECGs, but the money earmarked for it went to a fire truck instead. The paramedic union and medical control board were livid.) It was also an example of the ongoing friction between the two parties at some fire stations now overtly affecting provision of care to the public. It kicked off department infighting through the media, with the paramedic union becoming more militant in their demands for change. It also contributed to the Alberta Medical Association (AMA) threatening to stop providing medical control from

THE CALGARY FIRE DEPARTMENT ERA 1971–1984

emergency doctors, the only legal way for paramedics to perform certain life-saving procedures in the field. The AMA stated at the time that the province should create and fund a province-wide EMS system, something that wouldn't happen for another 20 years. The union created a list of concerns and recommendations, backed by the medical control board, and submitted them in confidence to the City. It was an unusual move for a union, said Paul Morck, treasurer for the union at the time, to push for standards and ask for recertification with ramifications for those who couldn't demonstrate their skills. They wanted to be proud of their profession, said Morck, and that meant raising the bar.

Somehow, the union's list of recommended changes made its way into the fire halls. The fire union wasn't happy and told their members to ostracize paramedics in the fire stations, for example no longer sharing meals with them. At Morck's station, he said there was a meeting led by the fire captain communicating this memo. Before the meeting was over, one firefighter rose, said, "Well, I've heard about enough. I've got to go make lunch for the paramedics," and walked away. He was soon followed by his colleagues. That's how it was in some fire halls—but not all. The relationships between the two halves tended to reflect whatever the fire captain felt about paramedics. If he liked them—things were good. But if not, it was a less friendly place for a paramedic.

Calgary City Council commissioned a report from a third party, Dr. Gerry Belton, a clinical psychologist, in 1982 to figure out what to do about the whole mess. Despite years of concerns about the organizational structure of the department, nobody had ever done a review of it. The Belton Report reviewed other EMS systems in Canada and the U.S. to see how they operated, either as part of a fire department or as a third service (in relation to fire and police) and surveyed local ambulance and fire staff. What Belton found wasn't surprising to people who worked in the department; it was like trying to mix oil and water in those fire halls.

Part of the report included getting input from members of fire and ambulance. In written survey responses, firefighters used terms like "glorified taxi drivers," "a Cadillac service," "playing doctor" and "superiority and arrogance" to describe their paramedic colleagues. On the other hand, paramedics wondered, "Why do I have to take orders from someone with only a St. John's certificate?" Belton found the firefighters had a clear culture, a paramilitary brotherhood that did not easily welcome outsiders. "When your life is on the line, your buddies will get you out," said one survey respondent when describing the firefighter ethos. The paramedic culture was more amorphous, Belton wrote, probably because it was still evolving as the job description and training had changed immensely over the past decade.[13]

In the end, Belton's report recommended essentially anything but the status quo organizational structure. In the current structure, it was unclear who was in charge of medical decisions at the site of an emergency. The report suggested three possible solutions: full integration and cross-training between fire and ambulance (where everyone would be trained as both a paramedic and a firefighter); total separation (i.e. the creation of a new emergency medical services department); or administrative separation (i.e. rebuilding the organizational structure of the fire department to address Ambulance Division concerns).

A task force made up of firefighters, paramedics, and union and City representatives took the Belton Report under advisement. Together they agreed the best solution was total separation of fire and EMS. They advised the creation of a new department and noted that continuing medical education and medical oversight would be key.

---

13 G.P. Belton. Organization Review Project. Report. Fire Department, Ambulance Division, City of Calgary. 1982.

THE NEW BOOMTOWN ERA
1984-1994

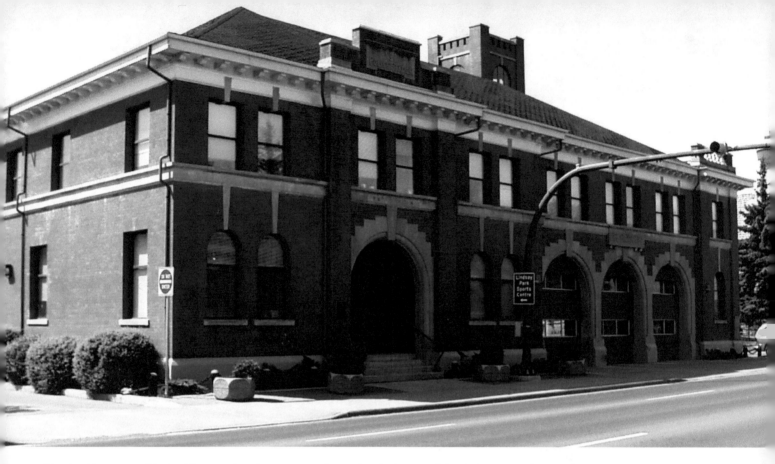

The first Emergency Medical Services headquarters was located in the former #2 fire hall near the Calgary Stampede grounds. The heritage building was nice-looking from the outside, but was overdue for renovation inside. (Courtesy of Bill McComb)

RAISING THE STAKES

On Jan. 1, 1984, "the divorce" was finalized. The Emergency Medical Services Department began operations at the City of Calgary, leaving behind their fire department roots. Sort of.

For all the recommendations suggesting physical separation would be beneficial for both departments, the economic reality was it was much easier to continue to house paramedics within fire halls. Fire stations continued to be shared spaces, only now the EMS Department was renting the space from the fire department. Most of the practical changes in the transition from division to department were administrative and managerial. Technically, it was a separate department.

THE NEW BOOMTOWN ERA 1984–1994

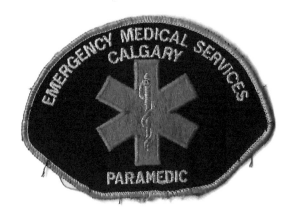

The new EMS Department came with a new shoulder crest in 1984. (Courtesy of Bill McComb)

It didn't always look like it, but it was starting to feel like it. Having a distinct line of command made for a significant shift in mentality for paramedics. Roles were more clearly defined at the fire hall and on the scene and morale was generally improved. There was still the odd fire captain at a hall who didn't get along with an individual paramedic or paramedics at large. Nobody's personality had changed, after all. Some firefighters felt a bit sore the EMS folks left them, making fire feel like they looked like the bad guys.

The EMS department was chasing the ambitious goal of having an all-ALS service. That would mean both medics who worked on an ambulance would be trained to the level of Emergency Medical Technician-Paramedic (EMT-P), the highest level of certification and able to provide advanced life support. Until they could get all staff to the paramedic level, each ambulance was required to have at least one EMT-P per ambulance; the other medic would be an EMT-A (the "A" is for "ambulance"), who was trained to provide basic life support.

A new EMS headquarters was created in the former #2 fire hall at Macleod Trail and 18th Avenue S.E. It wasn't exactly a shining beacon of a new future. The building was a provincial heritage resource originally built around the turn of the century to house both police and fire and by this point was home mostly to mice. In one supervisor's office, an ill-timed toilet flush would cause flooding in the floor below. His desk had to be propped up on one end because of the floor sinking from one side of the room to the other. But it was home. Shortly after moving in, the EMS inhabitants were moved out again so renovations could be done. Once it was more liveable, the historic fire hall served as EMS headquarters until 2005, when it was moved to the northeast community of Whitehorn.

One of the key recommendations for the newly created department was to install a director who was clearly in charge of the paramedics. Syd Cartwright was the first director of the new EMS Department. Cartwright came over from the City's planning department. Hiring an EMS outsider as boss was hard on morale at first. Cartwright was a strict disciplinarian. He had the tall task of

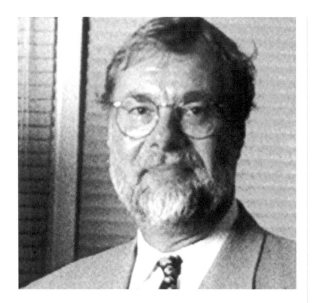

Syd Cartwright, first director of Calgary's EMS Department. (Courtesy of AHS EMS Archives)

holding the new department to a new standard of accountability and professionalism and he was laser-focused on that task. He was dealing with behaviour that would at times seem more suited to a frat house than an EMS operation: everything from pranks and firehall water fights to a paramedic who was found to be selling real estate out of the back of his ambulance.

In his first few years, Cartwright wasn't especially popular. So when a package arrived for him one day and a staff member noticed it was ticking, the staffer feared the worst. She called the police and in came the bomb squad.

The procedure to disrupt an explosive device was to douse the package in water to neutralize any sparks and counter an explosion. The bomb squad's robot approached the package, picked it up, and brought it to the front foyer of the evacuated building. It shot a jet of water forceful enough to blow a hole in the carpet. Only then was it safe to investigate the ticking package.

And that investigation revealed it was an antique pocket watch—now cracked on the face, but still ticking—later identified as a gift for Cartwright. Perhaps it was a sign of just how dire relations were that it seemed more likely for Cartwright to receive a bomb than a gift.

Along with a director, the new department required a medical director. The role of medical director had been unofficial until this point; now it was provincially legislated. Without a physician overseeing paramedic operations, an Alberta ambulance service could only provide horizontal transportation. Serendipitously, emergency medicine began developing as a specialty in the late 1970s. Up to that point in Calgary and most other places, emergency departments were staffed by general practitioners. These family doctors weren't necessarily experienced in dealing with trauma patients, but were required to work emergency department shifts to gain hospital privileges.

For medics, these emergency doctors were frequent purveyors of frustration as much as medicine. Because there had long been no or limited emergency training for these doctors, it was unpredictable what a doctor would tell a medic to do over the phone. The limited training wasn't ideal for patients, either. In a trauma situation, the doctor may not be able to do much more than triage a patient and hope they didn't get worse before a surgeon arrived.

As Calgary EMS Medical Director, Dr. Gil Curry's role was bridging that gap in the emergency medical system. After training in emergency medicine in Oakland, CA, and working closely with EMS there, Curry saw parallels between his work and what paramedics do. "We all like the adrenaline rush, especially when you know you can make a difference if you do things well," he said. He saw his job as supporting emergency doctors by giving paramedics formal guidelines to do their best work possible before they reached the hospital. He developed the first set of medical protocols for the department, widening Calgary paramedics' scope of practice, but within clear limits.

Before he could do his job, Curry had to win the respect of medics and other doctors. As a new specialty, emergency medicine needed to prove its worth. Curry credited Dr. Bob Johnson at the Calgary General Hospital for leading the emergency medicine charge and setting the bar high. On the other front, Curry had to demonstrate he wasn't just another doctor who thought paramedics were ambulance drivers who should drop patients off and get on their way—a view still held by some in the medical profession.

Early in his five years as medical director, Curry attended to a vehicle collision. A patient needed to be intubated at the scene while still in a vehicle. It's a really difficult position to provide aid in. Curry said he felt immense pressure to perform in that moment. He needed to show his EMS colleagues he could do more than sit and talk at someone's bedside. He did successfully intubate his patient and felt some of that weight lift off his shoulders. "Over time they had to accept I wasn't out to make their life worse," he said. "I made it very clear I was there to be there for the patient."

Curry's key contribution was developing the first set of medical protocols for Calgary EMS. The approximately 40 protocols were based on what the ambulance service used in Oakland, but specific to the Calgary context, like including the drugs that were allowed on Alberta ambulances. Alongside the protocols, the EMS Staff Development Division created continuing medical education for paramedics to keep them up to date with the at-times massive advances that had been made since paramedics had begun graduating in the early '70s. The bottom line of this training: train everyone to get better, not to penalize them if they weren't yet good enough. Every paramedic needed to prove their advanced life support skills in a two-day course every second year. Failure was frustrating. Paramedics who failed would no longer be in charge on their ambulance. But it kept standards high.

The protocols made clear, finally, what actions paramedics should and could take and when they needed to phone for medical control. There would be no more confusion, when someone's heart wasn't beating properly, about whether you were supposed to wait for a doctor to answer the phone. "Not having to patch on every critical patient really saved a lot of lives," said Paul Morck. It meant paramedics could defibrillate within seconds of getting to a cardiac patient instead of waiting minutes to get permission from a doctor. There's a saying that "time is brain." After about two minutes without oxygen, the brain and other organs reach a dangerous point of degradation. Between two and four minutes things drop off steadily and after four minutes function is lost precipitously. Similarly, humans, having a finite supply of blood, get into trouble very fast when it starts to leave their body. As the body tries to compensate by sending blood to protect its organs, it puts other tissue at risk. The sooner you can save that important tissue—like the brain—the better. Every second is precious.

Curry understood the exasperation paramedics felt with an unpredictable medical control system. He knew individual medics would respond to the same medical situations in different ways and that it could lead to taking the wrong action. A key piece of making the protocols practical was training for all the doctors who worked in emergency departments. Whoever picked up that call from a medic should understand what to do next. Curry's training for the doctors, backed by the medical control board, was mandatory, unpaid and not always popular. But it had an impact. Their results improved and those better results led to widening the scope of practice for paramedics over time. Curry said that laid the groundwork for what is today a "world-class service" in Calgary.

He served as medical director until 1990 when Dr. Peter Gant took on the role.

Under EMS Director Syd Cartwright was a paramedic named Tom Sampson. Sampson was a SAIT student doing his practicum on an ambulance in January 1984 when the new department was born. The following July he was hired into the EMS Department. Shortly after, the department learned the City would lose its contract for doing transfers between hospitals and from hospitals to nursing homes. (Transfers would instead be done by the Calgary District Hospital Group.) It was a big enough piece of the department's work that layoffs were expected amongst the staff. As a new guy, Sampson wanted to make himself less susceptible to a layoff and applied for a role in the department as a special projects co-ordinator in the lead-up to the 1988 Winter Olympics. He got it, despite being in the

THE NEW BOOMTOWN ERA 1984–1994

nascent years of his career. Half a year into that role, another opportunity came up. A big one. The department needed a new manager of operations and wanted every current manager and field superintendent to apply for the position. Sampson was intimidated by the prospect, but was compelled to apply. It wasn't just that he was nervous about another jump upwards so early in his career; the previous three managers of operations had only held the job for three, six and 11 months respectively. Nobody had been the right fit yet.

And then, at 29, he got the gig. "When I went into that job I had an incredible cadre of people there who were terribly experienced," said Sampson. "Some of those guys it felt like had 400 years of experience. It was tough.

"They were very good to me in terms of the way it was. But at the same time I had to become the manager, and part of the unit surviving was that we figured out how to work with Syd Cartwright."

Sampson said his job early on was to make the department more accountable, through new training and processes as well as showing evidence of that improvement. Training would now include demonstrating being able to execute the skills medics said they could do. Sampson also played buffer between Cartwright and staff. "Syd was incredibly powerful and incredibly opinionated about how he needed things to go," Sampson said.

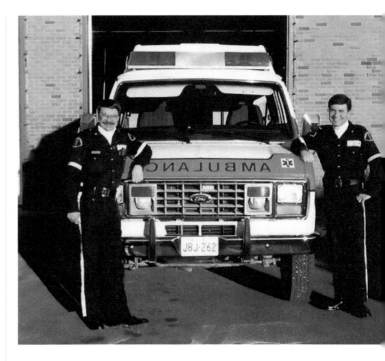

The one-piece jumpsuit uniform was designed to be easy to wear for those 2 a.m. calls that roused paramedics from sleep. They're modelled here, in 1987, by Bob Fisher and Bob Koloff. (Courtesy of Bill McComb)

67

MEDICAL ERRORS ARE BOUND TO HAPPEN

As the department aggressively pursued higher standards of medical care, the ability to treat more threatening things outside of the hospital became more available to Calgary paramedics. The overall level of patient care was increasing hugely, in large part due to the new medical protocols.

As Calgary's Emergency Medical Services became increasingly medical in nature, far surpassing its roots as horizontal transportation, medical errors were bound to occur. However, unlike in the health-care system, there was no precedent in the department for dealing with medical errors.

In 1987, two paramedics responded to a call concerning a hypoglycemic diabetic patient who had become combative. It was incredibly difficult for them to establish an IV—and on top of it the medics were working in low-light conditions. They hung a mini bag of what they thought was 250 ml of D5W—a 5% dextrose solution in water. In fact, it was D5W with 1,000 mg of lidocaine. While D5W treats a diabetic patient who is hypoglycemic, D5W with lidocaine is used in a cardiac event to stabilize the heart. The mistake happened because the labelling of the two bags was unclear—a small red line was all that differentiated the two. The drug error could have been fatal, but the patient didn't suffer any ill effects.

Medical errors have been happening as long as medicine has been practiced, but Syd Cartwright saw no place for it in his department. He directed Tom Sampson follow labour relations' advisement to suspend the paramedics who had responded to that call. Sampson was "shell-shocked," at the command, horrified that he was going to "ruin these guys, destroy their lives."

Dr. Gil Curry, too, was completely opposed to the suspensions. In Curry's view, paramedics had to feel safe and supported in reporting medical errors. Otherwise staff wouldn't come forward and that could mean bad things for patient care. He felt there needed to be systemic changes in training to fix these gaps, not punishment.

Cartwright was incensed that Curry opposed his direction and told him his services would no longer be required in the EMS Department. In fact, Curry's services were absolutely required. Without a medical director, the City couldn't provide paramedic services, only transportation to hospital.

Sampson considered quitting over the matter. He recalled being in tears when he told his two medics he had been directed to suspend them, making it clear he disagreed

THE NEW BOOMTOWN ERA 1984–1994

completely with the directive from above. It marked a turning point for the department. "It was pivotal in the sense that we needed to be accountable, but accountability, it didn't come without compassion," said Sampson. "If you've made an error when you're trying to do the very best with the best training that you have, that should be an opportunity to provide more education."

Both Curry and Sampson stayed in their positions as a new era began to unfold—one characterized by increased medical oversight and statistical analysis. An in-depth audit of the department was undertaken.

THE FITCH REPORT

The Fitch Report was a value-for-money audit executed by Fitch & Associates, one of the top consultants in the EMS field in North America. It resulted in close to 30 recommendations to bring Calgary EMS in line with the broader medical community through higher standards, including: an EMS-run dispatch system, using the Medical Priority Dispatch System, standardized medical protocols, a flexible deployment dispatch system to balance response times, a new radio system and generally elevated accountability.

One of the most wide-reaching Fitch recommendations was using the Medical Priority Dispatch System (MPDS). This was a system of protocols printed on 32 cardboard cards, for dispatchers to use to determine a patient's condition and what action to take next, including guiding the caller to take a medical intervention before the ambulance arrived if necessary. Calgary was the first in Canada to use MPDS, and by 1993, three years into using it, had been recognized as just the third service in the world to be called a "Centre of Excellence." In fact, it worked so well that a civilian working in dispatch with no medical training other than MPDS was able to help a father deliver a baby over the phone.

Key to making MPDS work was having an EMS-owned and operated dispatch centre. Dispatch centres around North America, if they were staffed by medics at all, tended to be staffed by medics who were injured or otherwise couldn't work on the street. Fitch recommended that Calgary's new dedicated dispatch centre be crewed by the best paramedics on the service. "We used to say the dispatch centre was the brain of the operations and the paramedics were the heart," said Paul Morck, who was Superintendent of Communications and implemented 19 of Fitch's recommendations.

Fitch also introduced a new approach to tracking and comparing ALS and BLS call data. It was the start of evidence-based decision-making. Crews didn't have formal criteria for what required advanced life support and what was basic—it was more about feeling whether they had provided significant care, said Dr. Peter Gant, medical director from 1990-98. Prior to Fitch's approach, Calgary EMS believed 50% of their calls required ALS care. After the criteria was specified (was the patient intubated? Did they require advanced life support such as intravenous medication? Did they require cardiac assistance such as CPR? Did they require a fluid bolus—a large amount of fluid in a short period of time?) they found only 15% of their calls required ALS

THE NEW BOOMTOWN ERA 1984–1994

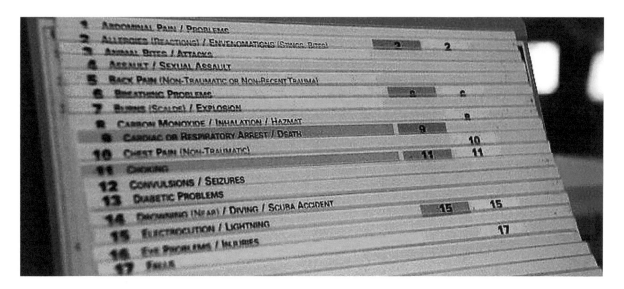

The Medical Priority Dispatch System was a game-changer, standardizing medical protocols over the phone. (Courtesy of AHS EMS Archives)

care and with a higher frequency of such calls in the downtown core. Flexible deployment was customized around this data with the understanding that response times needed to be quicker to ALS calls regardless of location. Fitch recommended a response time under eight minutes 90% of the time; Calgary EMS met that goal by the mid-1990s.

Flexible deployment was recommended to address uneven response time across the city. It was extremely unpopular amongst paramedics at first. Calgary had operated a fire department-style deployment. In that system, ambulance crews waited at their station until a call happened, then did the call, transported to a hospital and came home to the station. It meant a crew might have a night with no calls because nothing happened in their area of coverage, even if the rest of the city's medics were run off their feet and some citizens were waiting around for an ambulance.

Flexible deployment aimed to balance response times by sending units to another station for coverage while those units were out on a call. It meant better coverage for the city and that was better for patients, though it meant sacrificing downtime for paramedics. Gino Savoia recalled a night shift when he and his partner drove close to 300 km providing coverage without doing a single call. He acknowledged though that it made more sense than the old static deployment model, which was "ridiculous in hindsight." Later, the flexible deployment system was fine-tuned based on stats, mandating that coverage be provided at only particular stations where there had to be an ambulance available, like downtown. Over the years, with new computers and later GPS technology, the system was further refined and digitized.

The changes to dispatch—MPDS and flexible deployment especially—saved lives. There's no doubt about that. "Pre-alert" saved its fair share of lives, too. Pre-alert was a computerized process to immediately confirm an address and dispatch an ambulance. It shaved as much as 90 seconds off the time it took an ambulance to respond. When "time is tissue," that's all the time in the world.

The use of a computerized dispatch system didn't mean the manual system of the past was fully disregarded. If the computer system ever failed, there had to be a manual backup. So weekly, dispatch pulled out their cookie sheets. These were literally a series of maps glued onto cookie sheets used to track the location and status of ambulances using magnets. Those cookie sheets kept them sharp.

SIMMERING TOWARD A STRIKE

Despite the significant changes made in the short life of the Emergency Medical Services Department, paramedics were still struggling to find an identity in the city. In some ways, they still felt like the "poor cousins," particularly due to their pay being inferior to firefighters and police officers.

A decade before the department was created, it looked like the pay gap issue would be addressed when the paramedic union and the City were getting close to a new contract. But across the country in 1974, inflation had topped 10% per year (one of the effects of the OPEC oil crisis when oil prices quadrupled from US$3 to US$12 per barrel in mere months). Despite campaigning to the contrary, the federal government passed the Anti-Inflation Act in 1975, which limited wage increases on all businesses with at least 500 employees, as well as price controls. That move effectively derailed those paramedic contract negotiations and left the wage disparity to chafe all parties into the next millennium.

Paramedics wondered why they were getting paid less than firefighters with less training, but the same seniority. They were also unhappy with the use of paramedics working as EMT-As, which required just eight weeks of schooling compared to two years for a paramedic.[14] They were referred to as "taints," as in "it ain't a paramedic and ain't an EMT—you're neither." It was a budget decision that was loathed by staff.

Part of the reason behind the identity crisis for paramedics was that they straddled the two worlds of public service and medicine. "Nobody trusts us and nobody allows us to do the things that we were trained to do," said paramedic Claude Belobersycky. "It was a real challenge. We had to prove ourselves." Belobersycky said mistrust from outsiders had been part of the job at least since the ambulance service was part of the fire department. The public—most of who hadn't had direct experience with paramedics—didn't quite understand their role either.

Medical Director Dr. Peter Gant said that another sticking point at the time was mandated recertification for ALS skills for all medics. Gant said there was significant backlash because recertification was seen by some as an assault on their credibility.

---

14 Zimmerman, Kate. "Medics may Swap Life-Saving Duties for the Picket Line." *Calgary Herald*, April 1, 1990. https://search.proquest.com/docview/244058596?accountid=46584.

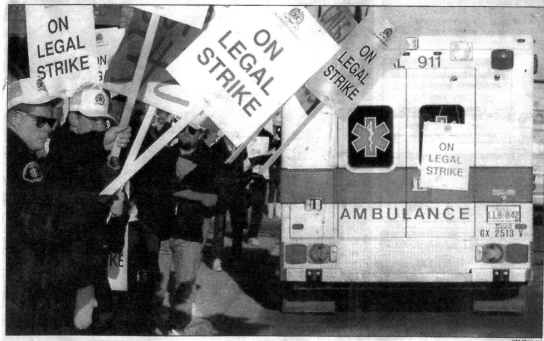

Calgary Sun Front Page Sunday, Dec. 15, 1991. (Courtesy of Postmedia News)

Calgary Sun Article Sunday Dec. 15, 1991. (Courtesy of Postmedia News)

ALL-OUT STRIKE

City insists public in good hands during labor stalemate: Page 3

PARAMEDIC PICKETS were out in force yesterday in front of Emergency Medical Services headquarters at Macleod Tr. and 18 Ave.

▼ LABOR

Paramedics begin full-scale walkout

By BILL KAUFMANN
Calgary Sun

Calgary's 177 paramedics began a full-blown strike yesterday for the first time in their history.

The paramedics walked off the job at noon, shortly after attempts to revive talks with the city failed.

No new negotiations are scheduled.

"As of this morning, there were eight units left and they've been removed as of today," said Richard Osborne, a spokesman for the Canadian Union of Public Employees Local 3421.

As he spoke, many motorists honked their support to dozens of pickets in front of Emergency Medical Services headquarters at Macleod Tr. and 18 Ave.

"I didn't expect the amount of noise we're hearing — it's a godsend," said Osborne.

"It keeps our morale up and lets the city administration know the public wants us treated fairly."

City officials are confident that a contingency plan whereby management operates ambulances — assisted by emergency physicians — will maintain the public's safety.

"Management are all trained paramedics who upgrade their skills every year," said city spokesman Marilyn Kaiser.

She said the normal 14 ambulances were on the road.

Kaiser said response time to calls was averaging the same as those of paramedics.

But union spokesmen say the managers are too few and they are ill-suited to ensure public safety.

"You have to be sharp and have skills.

"There are management people who haven't seen patients for as long as 12 years," said union spokesman Doug Odney.

"Some have never driven an ambulance in emergency situations."

Emergency dispatchers will determine priority life-threatening calls, said Kaiser, who urged those Calgarians with minor ailments to transport themselves to hospital.

"We just hope this is over with as soon as possible," she said.

The paramedics say they're close to accepting a wage settlement that gives them parity with city firefighters and a 13.5% pay hike over three years.

But they're upset with a city move to apply its own qualifications for paramedics' licensing instead of the existing provincial standards.

"The city has pushed and pushed. What they're saying is if we fail their course, we're not paramedics," said Odney.

Calgary's Voice

KEN M. KING, Publisher
CRAIG MARTIN, Associate Publisher
MARIO SGROI, General Manager
ROBERT POOLE, Editor-in-Chief
PAUL JACKSON, Editor
CHRIS NELSON, Managing Editor

Audit Bureau of Circulations Member

November paid circulation 70,270

J. DOUGLAS CREIGHTON, Chairman of the Board and CEO
PAUL V. GODFREY, President and COO   BRUCE L. JACKSON, Vice-President Finance and CFO

The Calgary Sun, a division of the Toronto Sun Publishing Corporation, is published at 2615 12 Street N.E., Calgary, Alberta, T2E 7W9.

Cheated

CALGARY'S PARAMEDICS acted in good faith when they voted to accept a new contract and returned to work.

But now they have been slapped in the face and had the rug pulled from under them by the eight aldermen who voted to veto the proposed contract.

This is an absolute disgrace — and the paramedics have a right to be both furious and bitter.

And it's incredible that after suddenly vetoing the offer made by the city's negotiating team, council members would be so naive as to believe paramedics would cheerfully remain on the job.

But in voting 12 to 2 to ask that paramedics not walk out, aldermen demonstrated total blindness to the situation.

The paramedics, after all, had been told they had a deal subject to what they thought was a simple technicality of ratification.

Then suddenly, they learned that in the eyes of eight aldermen, a deal is not necessarily a deal.

Now, how can we expect other unions to approach negotiations believing the city's negotiating team has any real power to sign on the dotted line?

No, council has set the scene for future negotiations to be conducted amidst an atmosphere of suspicion and distrust.

It's said that aldermen backed off from the deal because they'd been hearing from voters that the 13.5% wage increase over three years was too generous considering the economic times.

If so, why didn't council set better parameters for its negotiating team?

Here at the *Sun* we don't believe in strikes.

We think they are outmoded, and there are better ways to settle labor disputes.

But just this once, we can understand why the paramedics are off the job.

Calgary Sun Editorial Wednesday, Jan. 8, 1992. (Courtesy of Postmedia News/Provided by Tom Sampson)

All these issues were simmering leading up to November 1991 when 12 paramedics working in dispatch went on strike. They'd been working to rule, including refusing to pull billing reports during midnight shifts. After one of their colleagues, Gino Savoia, was suspended indefinitely for his refusal to pull the reports, the picket line began. By Dec. 14, all 177 city paramedics were striking.

To keep EMS operating during the strike, ambulances were staffed by other department employees, including EMS administration and supervisors (who were all paramedics), plus Calgary Transit supervisors (who drove the ambulances) and emergency room doctors and nurses. It pushed emergency physicians way out of their comfort zones, said Gant. But it also gave them a whole new perspective on what it was to be a paramedic. "It allowed them to see what these ALS providers have to deal with in an out-of-hospital environment," said Gant. Post-strike, that appreciation was healthy for the relationship between the physicians and EMS. Gant said they enjoyed a honeymoon period for a while after that, which was good for patients, too.

EMS supervisors and doctors were working exhausting 24- and 36-hour shifts and the media covered the strike closely. Even the *Calgary Sun*, whose editorial board wasn't particularly fond of unions in general, published their support for the paramedics and criticism of city council's failure to strike a deal.

The union and the City finally sat down to talk, wanting to make a deal before Christmas. They came out with what seemed a fair deal, that included pay parity with firefighters, and would be ratified by city council after Christmas break. The paramedics ended their strike on Dec. 23 and went back to work.

But then city council utterly shocked paramedics by rejecting their own offer shortly after New Year's. It was unprecedented. The paramedics walked out again on Jan. 6. The night before the walkout, paramedics drove their ambulances onto the steps of the city municipal building, turned on their emergency lights, locked the doors and left. An ice fog over the city that night made for an eerie image. Perhaps it was an apt symbol of darker feelings this time around. During this second strike, paramedics responded to calls, but unless they were with a patient, they locked the ambulance and considered themselves off-duty.

When supervisors attempted to access ambulances to respond to calls, they were rebuffed. Paul Morck was one of those supervisors. Along with his management colleagues and doctors, they had enough staff to get four ambulances on the street. Typically, the ambulance bays were not locked, but that day they were. Morck had come over from dispatch where he'd just taken a call from a distressed woman whose husband had had a heart attack she had begged Morck to send an ambulance. Morck was distraught over being told at mechanical services that he wasn't able to access the ambulances, which were behind a locked garage door. Morck wasn't going to wait around. He ripped part of the man door off its hinges with his bare hands and tossed his fellow management paramedic through the opening. They now had access to the ambulances.

Within two days, the City had sweetened the pot, offering more than they had in the first round (the contract aldermen had rejected at the last minute). "It really was bizarre," chief negotiator Tom Chesterman told the *Calgary Herald* at the time. "The only analysis we can make is that either council is incredibly stupid or there's a miscommunication between administration and council."[15] From Claude Belobersycky's perspective, the strike made a huge difference to public perception and made a dent in the constant battle to prove how important their role was.

---

15 Ferguson, Eva. "Council Shot itself in Foot, Say Paramedic Leaders." *Calgary Herald*, Jan. 12, 1992. https://search.proquest.com/docview/244137407?accountid=46584.

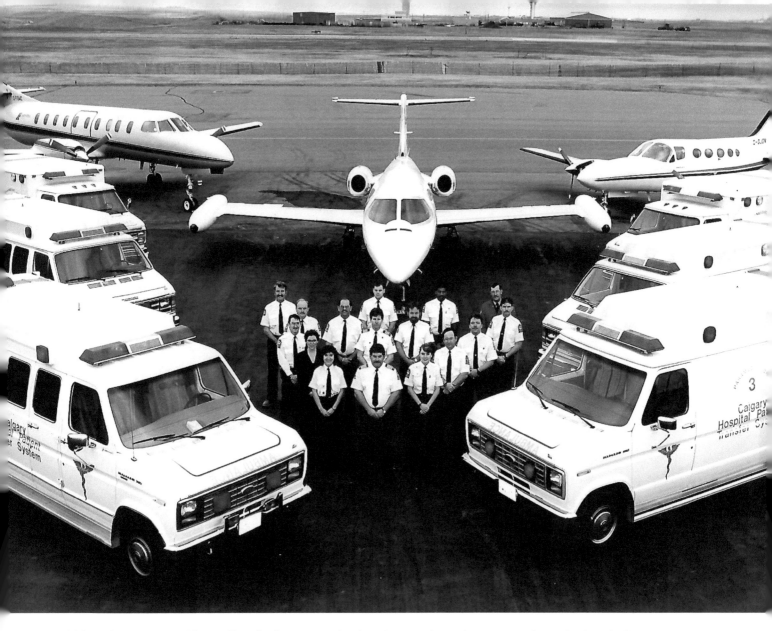

In 1986 the Calgary Hospital Patient Transfer System was developed as an independent program devoted to inter-facility transport. Initially operated by the Calgary District Hospital Group and subsequently the Calgary Regional Health Authority, it was absorbed into AHS EMS in 2009. (Courtesy of AHS EMS Archives)

VITAL SIGNS

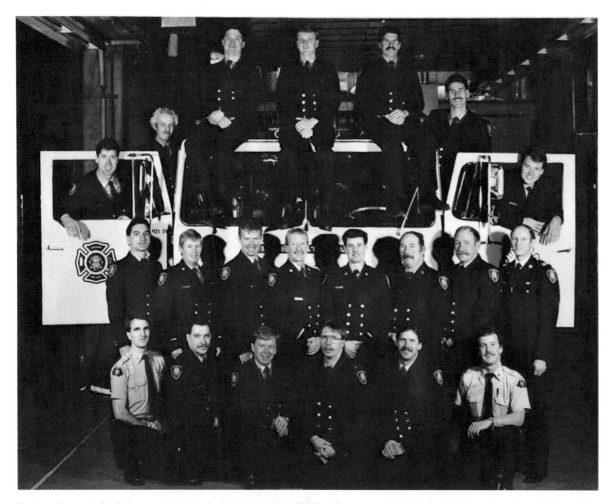

Paramedics and firefighters coexisting happily in the late 1980s. (Courtesy of Bill McComb)

FENDING OFF FIRE

The shared spaces of the fire halls were uncomfortable in the spring of 1992. The strike action hadn't helped. There was a feeling in the fire department that the strike was unprofessional. History looked like it would repeat itself when a task force was formed to make a plan to house EMS

THE NEW BOOMTOWN ERA 1984–1994

services within the fire department, yet again categorizing ambulance staff as fire civilians rather than cross-training all members in an integrated service to be firefighter paramedics. There was a small group within the EMS Department that liked the idea of working within the fire department, imagining higher wages and no more of that hectic flexible deployment model. (There was a joke amongst paramedics that a firefighter's two day shifts and two night shifts rotation was "two picnics, two sleepovers and four days off." Better fire suppression technology meant fewer fire calls, after all.) Mostly, the feeling from paramedics was that going back to the fire department days would be a step backward. Tom Sampson said it felt like he was always on alert holding back the fire department from taking over EMS. From his view, it was never because anyone believed that merging the departments was the best thing for patient care. Rather, it seemed driven by the fire union of the day, who saw more work for firefighters if they were part of the paramedic response.

The closest the two sides came to remarrying was in 1994. A merger had been proposed that would see all medics cross-trained as firefighters (it was decided that was simpler than training firefighters to be paramedics) and, importantly, would ensure every second person promoted to fire captain had to be a paramedic. That was to ensure that if the fire captain was going to be the lead at a medical scene, they were medically trained.

That particular battle came to a head in late February 1994 at a city council committee meeting. The meeting was ostensibly a chance for the council committee to review the proposal for merging the departments. Yet, when the meeting was about to start, City administrators distributed a press release announcing forthcoming changes—despite the plan not being reviewed, studied or approved by council. The council committee took major exception to this assumption by administration and killed the proposal by miring it in further studies and review.

That wasn't the end of the "will they, won't they" with the fire department. The constant question was a distraction from training, doing their jobs and contributing to the paramedical field, said Sampson. All the same, he said his staff did incredible work. "I don't think medics… truly understood what a significant impact they had on people's lives and how just incredible (they are)."

Finally, in 2005, Sampson had clear proof that his department would be left alone (by the fire department, at least). Sampson asked new Fire Chief Bruce Burrell flat out if Burrell was planning to take over EMS. Burrell told him he wasn't, not even if the two of them were holding hands at city hall. Sampson took that back to his staff and told them it was time to let go of the baggage that had been weighing them down for so long.

VITAL SIGNS

New Alberta Premier Ralph Klein really wanted to pay off the province's deficit and debt. The province had, in 1992, the highest deficit per capita in Canada, and Klein's popularity allowed him to rally Albertans behind his austere approach. Ralphonomics meant making deep 20% cuts across the entire public spending budget. It hit the health-care budget hard. One of the ways it manifested was creating a regional health authority system of 17 health regions across the province, replacing hospitals' individual boards, which often overspent their budgets. The new Calgary Regional Health Authority (CRHA) became the overseer of all city hospitals. Immense restructuring happened across the health-care system, including moving patients and programs, specializing hospitals and closing beds.

And then came the decision to blow up one of Calgary's oldest and most beloved hospitals.

THE HALLWAY
MEDIC ERA
1994-2009

Thousands of Calgarians gathered on surrounding hills to watch the Calgary General Hospital be demolished. For some, it was simply a thrilling implosion. For many in the medical community, it was the exclamation mark on heartbreak. (Courtesy of AHS EMS Archives)

THE HALLWAY MEDIC ERA 1994–2009

A HOSPITAL IMPLOSION AND A POPULATION EXPLOSION

The Calgary General Hospital was deemed too old and too expensive to update by 1994.[16] At least, that was the stance from the Calgary Regional Health Authority. Physicians and citizens who loved the General disagreed. Those who wanted to save the General[17] considered it to be an important part of the local health-care system, not just for the beds that existed there, but for its accessible location near the downtown of a growing city and its exceptional staff. "You could count on the old General to handle anything you sent at them," said Bill McComb. He recalled one day when the hospital was running three Code 99s—cardiac resuscitations—simultaneously with the help of paramedics. "They never turned anyone down. 'Just come on in.'"

Despite vocal concerns from medical professionals and the public, including producing studies that offered alternatives, the Calgary General Hospital was closed and its programs and staff transferred to other local hospitals. First, the emergency department was shuttered in 1996, then the rest of it in 1997. In October 1998, all eyes in the city turned to the General as it was demolished.

---

16 Alberts, Sheldon. "Bow Valley Grapples with its Demise: Controversy Swirls Around the Planned Demise of Calgary's Bow Valley Centre, Popularly Known as the General Acute Care Crisis." *Calgary Herald*, July 13, 1996. https://search.proquest.com/docview/244518856?accountid=46584.

17 The General was rechristened the Bow Valley Centre of the Calgary General Hospital in 1988 after merging with the Peter Lougheed Centre of the Calgary General Hospital. But it's best remembered by the name it had worn since it was just a two-storey wood-frame house on the banks of the Bow River in 1890.

Dust particles obscured the city skyline as the hospital—some of its seven buildings newer than the Foothills and Rockyview—crumbled.

"All the serious calls that we had in the downtown core, the stabbings, the overdoses, the fights in the bars, the traumas that we had, would go to the General Hospital," said Tom Sampson. "The General staff had a can-do attitude that was remarkable. They say that a facility is a place to go, but sometimes the people are really what made it. The staff at the General were legendary for their capacity to care for the people in the core. That's what it lost when they blew it up."

The Holy Cross Hospital in south downtown was similarly closed before being sold, as was the Grace Hospital in Hillhurst.

Ostensibly, these closures would help the province erase its debt, but blowing up a hospital doesn't do anything to change the number of patients in a city. It was a turning point for health care in Calgary. Calgary would be the only major centre in Canada without a significant hospital in the downtown core. At the same time, Calgary was growing fast and far out. The city's population had more than doubled from 385,000 in 1970, to 790,498 in 1997. The edges of the city were expanding and those suburbs were filling up, putting more demands on ambulance response times and hospital wait times alike. Around the early 1990s, Calgary EMS had rules mandating that an ambulance crew had to be in and out of the hospital, including doing their paperwork, in 20 minutes. Those 20-minute turnarounds were about to become a relic.

After the announcement of the hospital closures, but before they actually happened, the Foothills Hospital was designated the sole trauma centre for the city. While other emergency departments would operate at the Rockyview and Lougheed hospitals, all ambulances with traumatically injured patients would be transported to Foothills. Aligning with that move, that hospital became the central location for neurosurgery, orthopedics, heart surgery and internal surgery.

Just a week after the General's emergency department was closed and the new sole trauma centre system began, it was shoved into the media spotlight. A major traffic collision occurred two kilometres from the Peter Lougheed Centre. A teen driver with three teen passengers was driving to work when he collided with a city bus. Careening toward a home, the bus uprooted a tree before stopping at the doorstep.[18] Three of the car's critically injured occupants needed to be transported to Foothills—13 km away. A STARS air ambulance helicopter may have been called in if there were anywhere to land it. Instead,

---

18 Mario Toneguzzi, Mark Lowey and, Monte Stewart. "Crash Sparks Health Questions: Injured Shuttled to Foothills from N.E." *Calgary Herald*, April 15, 1997. https://search.proquest.com/docview/244587257?accountid=46584.

THE HALLWAY MEDIC ERA 1994–2009

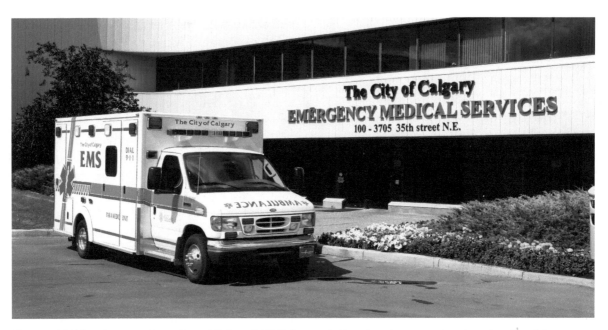

The new EMS headquarters in northeast Calgary's Whitehorn neighbourhood was spacious, housing dispatch, emergency management and Calgary Police Services as well. (Courtesy of AHS EMS Archives)

police dispersed down 16th Avenue, closing a dozen intersections from one side of the city to the other. The ambulances blazed lights and sirens to the hospital in five minutes.

Two of the teens died of their injuries. Immediately, the teens' families, the public and the media questioned whether the single trauma centre approach made sense in Calgary and wondered why the boys couldn't have been brought to the Lougheed instead. Officials explained that the emergency department at the Lougheed wouldn't have been able to attend to their extensive injuries. They said it was better to have a very good centralized trauma centre rather than dispersing resources around the city. An op-ed in *The Globe and Mail*[19] following the collision said that Calgarians had been generally supportive of the Klein government's austerity. Until that moment. "They have started some rather black jokes about how we'd all better plan our car accidents in the right quadrant of the city—the

---

19 Mitchell, Alanna. "Accident Cuts Deeply into Matter of Faith." *The Globe and Mail*, April 18, 1997. https://search.proquest.com/docview/384865378?accountid=46584.

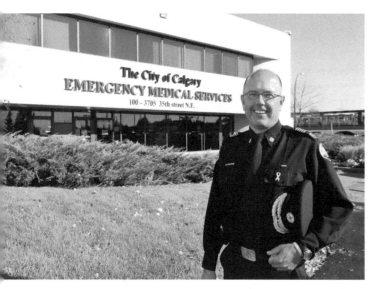

Tom Sampson, Chief, EMS. (Courtesy of AHS EMS Archives)

northwest—where the trauma centre is," wrote Alanna Mitchell.

Today, centralized trauma care is recognized as the optimal approach. Putting all the best professionals into one place where they attend to the same kinds of trauma regularly means they're better at treating it than someone who only sees that trauma three times a year. The nature of Calgary as a city means there are long transportation distances to the Foothills from the north or south edge of the city, but as long as people need emergency departments, there's always going to be some distance to travel. In 2018, Foothills was the busiest trauma centre in Canada because of the centralized approach and because it serves not just Calgary, but also much of southern Alberta.

STARS Air Ambulance is a critical part of patient transport in a sprawling Calgary today. The helicopter can be the difference between life and death when someone is critically injured—particularly at rush hour anywhere far from the Foothills hospital. Bill McComb recalled an incident at the Foothills Industrial Park, which, despite its name, is nowhere near the hospital. A man was spray painting in a sea can when his paint spray hit a halogen work light and exploded. He was critically burned. STARS was called to land in an adjacent parking lot. The ambulance crew packed him in and STARS was able to transfer him to the Foothills in around five minutes. McComb estimated that a ground trip, at best, would take 15 minutes, and more likely more than 20 minutes.

Tom Sampson succeeded Syd Cartwright as director of EMS in 1997, taking on the new title of Chief, EMS. His vision was to create an identity for the department, which included updated branding featuring the star of life on ambulances and the uniform. Sampson said adding professionalism and processes created an identity, and with that came pride in the work. Their new ambulances, high quality and expensive units, made for ever-better "offices" for medics.

The department purchased protective bulletproof vests to keep medics safe in the

THE HALLWAY MEDIC ERA 1994–2009

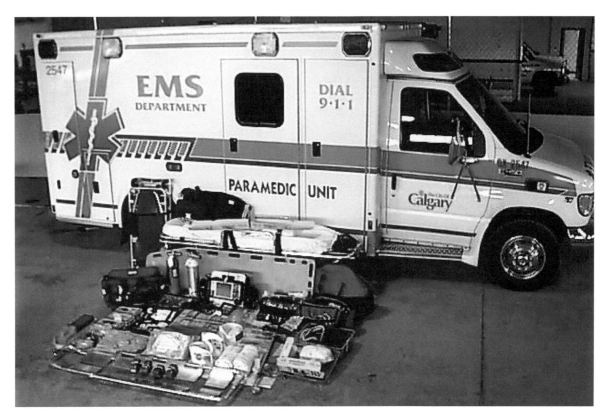

Modular ambulances—and the equipment they carried—in the late 1990s had come a long way from their counterparts just 30 years earlier. (Courtesy AHS EMS Archives)

field in 1998. It's an unpredictable, job, after all. "You never know what a day's going to bring in this job," said Claude Belobersycky, who once helped a mother deliver her baby during a garage sale. "You see things in that job that the average person would not see in a lifetime." It was a leap forward from the old days when medics didn't yet wear gloves to protect against blood-borne illness. "Back then, the more blood you got on you, the cooler it was. We look back now and go, 'Wow, what were we thinking?'"

At the same time, Calgary's neighbourhoods were growing so rapidly that the City could barely keep their maps up to date. There was a time when ambulances were stocked with maps that were updated annually. By

VITAL SIGNS

1999, they needed maps updated almost weekly. In one publicized case, an ambulance took 20 minutes to respond to a call because they couldn't find the location—it turned out a street name had been changed since their maps were last issued.

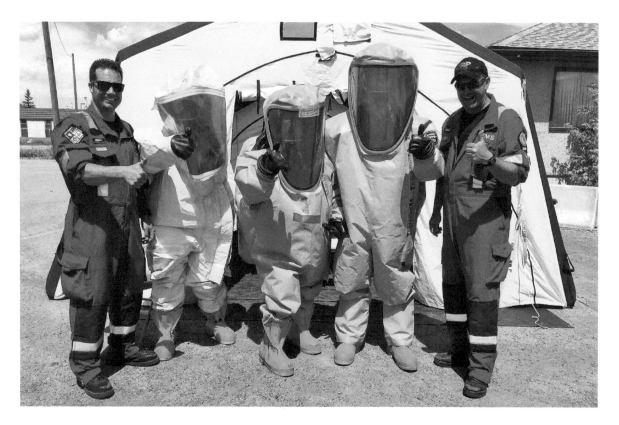

Incident Response Paramedics need to be prepared for any kind of contamination—as their suits suggest. (Courtesy of AHS EMS Archives)

THE ERA OF PARAMEDIC SPECIALIZATION

In October 2001, a tragic accident during a police training exercise kicked off a series of events that would influence a program that has saved multiple lives. Const. Darren Beatty was training with the Calgary Police Tactical Unit when he was fatally shot during a training exercise. The police service was rocked by the horrendous mishap. Prior to joining the police and the police TAC team, Beatty had spent four years as a paramedic. In his role with the police, he envisioned a tactical EMS program. While the Calgary Police tactical team had been in place since Black Friday in 1974, there was no EMS equivalent, nor a medic member on the police TAC team.

THE HALLWAY MEDIC ERA 1994–2009

In addition to Beatty's vision, a few incidents in the preceding years pointed to the need for Calgary to have a tactical EMS unit that could work with the police in high-risk situations. For example, in June 1999, a Calgary police member's leg was crushed in a vehicle by a suspect who was trying to evade arrest. The officer suffered in pain for 20 minutes before paramedics could attend to them. In 2001, Police Chief Jack Beaton committed to creating a Tactical EMS (TEMS) unit as a legacy for Const. Beatty.

The TEMS application process and training is gruelling. The physical and psychological assessments were modelled after Calgary police tactical operations. They include: high-angle rescue training for scaling buildings; skid training on the outside of a helicopter; dealing with clandestine drug labs; specialty munitions training, including disarming police guns; forced entry; using explosives; officer rescue; plus the kinds of injuries to expect in the role and how to establish a safe distance from a dangerous police operation. Brian Boechler was a paramedic-turned-police-officer when he applied to TEMS. He said the training required a police mindset that was outside the norm for most paramedics at the time. For example, quitting was not an option, Boechler said. That meant if you were running and couldn't take another step, you better start to crawl. It wasn't just about how good you were at a skill, but how well you worked with others and how much trust you could build.

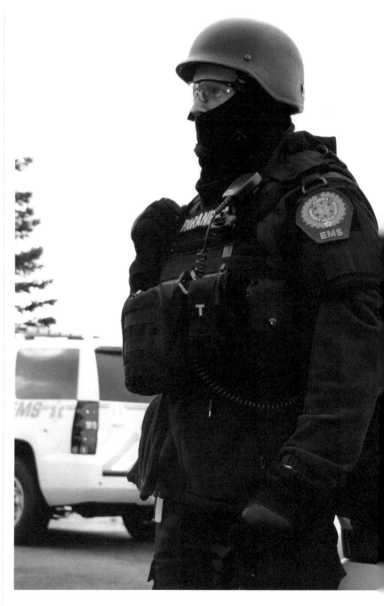

Tactical paramedic. (Courtesy of AHS EMS Archives)

Twelve paramedics made it through the application process to go through full training. By the end, the tactical paramedics were prepared for work in an extreme police environment. While all paramedics are trained to treat, for example, a gunshot wound, a tactical paramedic has expanded training to deal with incidents where they're unable to extract a patient for rapid transport and need to treat them at the scene for an extended period. Just as important, the police unit uses extremely specialized tactics. In certain circumstances, throwing a paramedic into a high-risk incident without knowledge of those tactics could cause harm, said Boechler.

TEMS paramedics work their regular paramedic rotation in addition to being deployed with the Calgary Police Service's elite TAC team. When they're on scene with the TAC unit, the tactical paramedic's top priority is injured officers, followed by any suspect who may be injured.

Doug Odney, the first superintendent for the TEMS unit and now commander of Calgary's 9-1-1 Centre, said having tactical paramedics in Calgary has undoubtedly saved life and limb. In March 2018, Const. Jordan Forget was one of several officers to respond to a call for a home break-in right on the heels of an armed robbery and an attempted carjacking. When officers descended upon the suspect, the suspect opened fire, with police returning shots. That's when Forget was shot in the chest with a rifle round. Odney notes that there was a tactical medic onsite who was able to immediately attend to Forget, who had a collapsed lung.

"For me, it was very, very emotional there to see how that event went," said Odney. "It truly shows the impact of what happens sometimes to police officers in the line of duty… it shows the value of those services because sometimes people take it for granted."

As the city grew, EMS developed more specialized groups and response protocols to meet its needs. Starting in 2000, Calgary's hazardous materials medics worked alongside the fire department at scenes with environmental contamination. They were there to help patients who might also have toxic materials on them, like a gas or chemical spill or fumes. These patients would then be transported to the hospital, but there was always a risk of cross-contamination from the incident. So, over the years, the response was refined and developed into a specialized Incident Response Paramedic role, who are also known as IRPs.

IRPs respond to calls where the scene or patient is believed to have any kind of hazardous contamination, including chemical, biological, radiation, nuclear or environmental. Whether it's the threat of carbon monoxide or suspicious white powder, they're prepared. Typically, IRPs work in pairs. In fact, the specialized protective suits they wear at the scene require another person's help to put on

THE HALLWAY MEDIC ERA 1994–2009

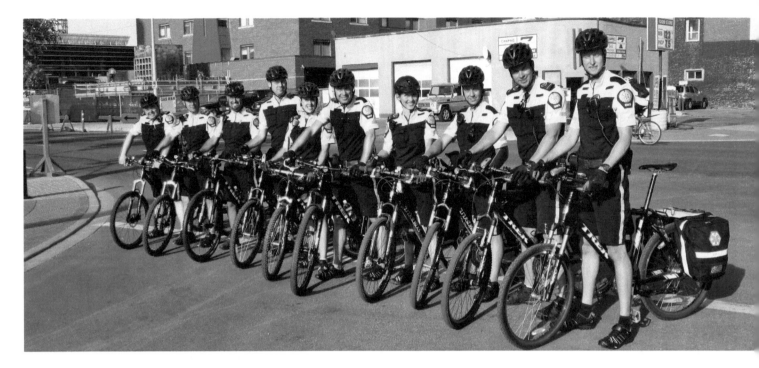

Rapid Access Paramedics. (Courtesy of AHS EMS Archives)

and remove. These paramedics are experts in hazardous materials and will be called to diverse scenes, from the disassembly of a meth lab or a train derailment to a commercial building fire or an airplane emergency.

Key to the IRP's role is decontamination of patients. In one case, a patient had become saturated in gasoline due to a vehicle's gas line rupture. While he wasn't injured, he did need to be assessed in hospital and it was extremely risky to move him before cleaning off all the gasoline.

Around the mid-1990s, Calgary EMS took over medical services at the Calgary Police arrest processing unit (APU) downtown. Every fresh arrest that came in had to have a medical assessment, said Bob "Bullet" Willis, who worked the unit. In the early days, there would be just one paramedic on an overnight shift, which got extremely busy. Willis said he at times had 120 people to assess on a single shift, before staffing was adjusted to account for the amount of work. Willis also set up a student program at the APU to give SAIT students

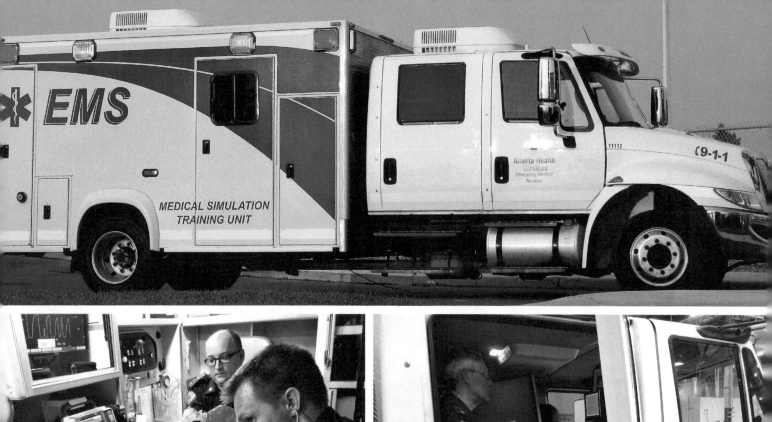

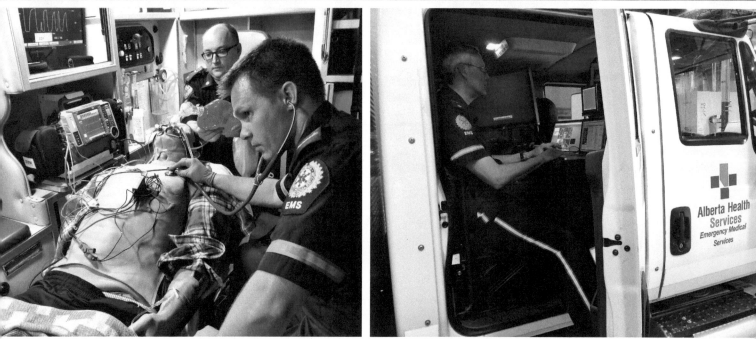

Medical Simulation Training is an incredibly realistic way to mimic real-life medical emergencies. The crew undergoing training must react to the life-like symptoms controlled by the trainer operating the simulation. The mobile unit can bring training to crews around the province. (Courtesy of AHS EMS Archives)

some eye-opening, hands-on experience. He said he definitely scared off some students, but he's practical about it. "You need head and hands to be a paramedic," he said.

Another team, Rapid Access Paramedics, roll into action in totally different circumstances. The bike-riding medics are the people poised on scene where there are large crowds like music festivals, the Calgary Stampede Parade and marathons. Modelled on the police service's mountain bike units, they carry all their first response equipment on their bikes so that they can get to patients in places where navigating an ambulance to them wouldn't be feasible. Key to their success is their ability to assess a patient and communicate whether they need further care, especially at a chaotic, loud or unpredictable outdoor event.

The spring of 2004 saw the RAP team in a particularly lively environment on 17th Avenue South when the Calgary Flames made a run in the Stanley Cup Playoffs. With the avenue's proximity to both the Saddledome and dozens of bars and restaurants where fans were watching the games, it was packed. It became the "Red Mile," with thousands of people celebrating in the street, many of them having had plenty to drink over the course of the game (and perhaps the hours leading up to it). The RAP team could navigate the jersey-clad crowds and respond and triage as needed.

The City placed a priority on training their medics to keep their skills up and aligned with medical advances. In the early 2000s, Calgary became the first service to use patient care simulation for pre-hospital care training. The goal with patient care simulation is to emulate a real environment as closely as possible and recreate situations that are either common for the medic but need to be improved upon, or high-acuity, low opportunity events. The latter skills need to be razor sharp to save lives. The computer-operated simulated patient can speak, make bodily noises and present whatever symptoms are required to mimic a real situation. Based on how the medics act, their patient will stabilize or deteriorate. They can see their patient's ECG results, oxygen saturation, blood pressure, pulse and more. It allows the paramedics to practice—and make mistakes—without harm to a real person. Today, there are three mobile training units used around the province, plus a new medical flight simulator to train medics and other health professionals to work on fixed-wing crafts.

VITAL SIGNS

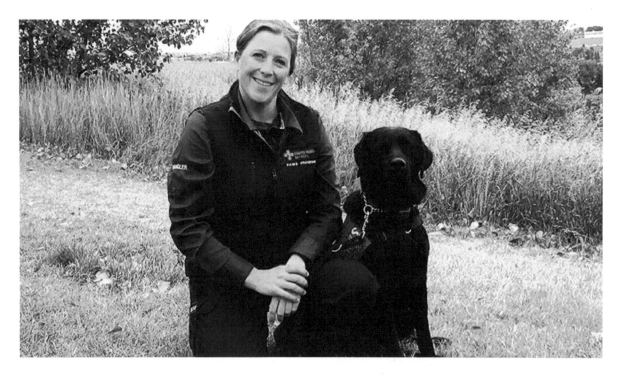

Erica Olson, an Advanced Care Paramedic, and her canine colleague Delray help in debriefings following critical incident stress events. It's the first program of its kind in North America. (Courtesy of AHS EMS Archives)

THIS JOB TAKES ITS TOLL

People who respond to emergency situations see a different version of our world. It's a view without the filter of a newspaper reporter or TV camera, the thoughtful crop of a photojournalist or careful wording of a historian. Being on the scene of a tragedy is a visceral experience. Until the mid-1990s, there wasn't much formal mental health support for Calgary's ambulance attendants and later paramedics. It's one of those jobs, like police and fire, where there's a perception that the people who go into the job have accepted the difficult nature of it and that somehow because of that they shouldn't complain. Paramedics were more or less left to deal within their own support system.

Ron Firth, who worked as an ambulance attendant in 1970, then trained and worked as a paramedic until retiring as a superintendent in 2004, looks back with some regret on the lack of support for traumatic situations early in his career.

"If everybody's killed, there's nothing you can do. It takes a toll on you, too. The more of these bad calls you go to, the more stress is going to be on you." He said nobody talked about critical incident stress or post-traumatic stress during his time in the field. "You just had to sort of basically forget about the call and go on with your life. That's the only way you survived. If you start worrying about every call where you've had a bad experience, it's going to eat you alive."

Bill McComb credited his wife for helping him through countless calls. Such a call happened one winter in the 1970s, when McComb was in his mid-20s. His crew was sent to the shores of the Bow River in Inglewood to pick up the body of an eight-year-old boy who had drowned. The scene was just a few blocks from McComb's home where he lived on the riverbank with his wife and young son. "Police divers had recovered the boy's body and laid it in the snow on the bank. Close by was a solitary set of small footprints leading to a hole in the ice. The boy's arms were crossed over his chest, his cheeks were puffed out and his eyes were squeezed tight shut; he had died," McComb wrote.

"When I arrived home that evening, my wife was quite shocked when I grabbed our young son, gave him a shake and a tight hug and then proceeded to tell him in no uncertain terms that he was not to go near the river without an adult present. Then, as in many incidents over the years, I was able to talk with my wife about the experience and get her perspective and support, which enabled me to deal with the stress."

By the late 1990s, the City of Calgary's EMS Department was a leader in Canada in Critical Incident Stress Management. Critical incident stress is a precursor to PTSD; PTSD usually results from the accumulation of several critical incidents when they're not dealt with by the individual in a healthy timeframe. Calgary EMS's Critical Incident Stress Management's now-long-standing program is a peer-to-peer program intended to support medics within 48 hours of a critical incident. It's generally face to face and can be one on one or in a group setting. Staff can request CISM anytime they need support debriefing.

On a difficult call, partners can be there for one another to debrief in an informal way, but the CISM approach allows a neutral peer to come in and talk through it.

In its current form, CISM Peer Support also aims to help medics build resiliency by offering support and additional resources and making sure they know they're not alone in having strong feelings about a particular call. In 2015, AHS EMS established a psychological

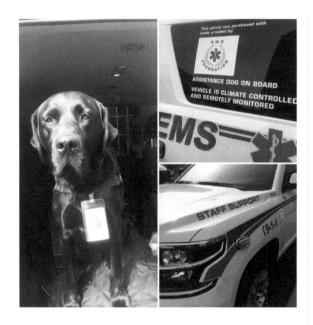

Delray and Paramedic Erica Olson travel in an EMS response vehicle donated by the EMS Foundation. The Chevy Tahoe is equipped to respond to emergencies, including those where patient transport may not be necessary. (Courtesy of AHS EMS Archives)

In 2017, the Psychological Awareness and Wellness Support program, called PAWS, launched. With the support of the EMS Foundation, Delray, a trained canine therapy dog, travels the province. Along with his paramedic handler Erica Olson, Delray helps out in debriefings for critical incident stress events and provides day-to-day stress management. Olson is an Advanced Care Paramedic with mental health support training. Together, they're offering the first service dog program directed specifically at the mental health of EMS providers in North America. Currently, PAWS is in the midst of an 18-month trial program. If it's deemed successful, the plan is to expand PAWS throughout the five AHS zones across the province.

McComb was a field superintendent and a grandfather when he attended a fatal CTrain collision. A woman was driving a truck with her elderly mother and young daughter in the vehicle with her when she turned and drove in front of a CTrain at 36th Street N.E.. The CTrain car was derailed, causing several minor injuries inside. The woman's mother was killed and she and her daughter injured.

health committee. Their goal is to understand and improve the care of medics' psychological health during and after critical incidents, as well as the burden of day-to-day work life. Part of that includes a mental health program modelled after the Canadian Department of National Defense. Supervisors and peer support teams are now trained in applied suicide intervention skills. CISM workers receive formal training and 24/7 counselling support is available for EMS practitioners.

"It was a major call with lots of triage and supervision involved," McComb wrote. "When all the ambulances had left the scene, transporting to various hospitals around the city, I suddenly found myself all alone with my emotions. I ended up parked at the side of the road somewhere away from the scene of the crash, trying to control my tears when Tom Sampson phoned me about an unrelated issue. I answered the phone, but was unable to talk. He quickly understood the situation and shortly thereafter, I got a call from a CISM Peer Support person (a fellow superintendent) who simply talked with me on the phone and helped me resolve my feelings."

Paramedic Carolyn Kremer said different calls can have particular impact based on a medic's personal life. She recalled responding to a fatal car accident involving a woman who was four months pregnant while Kremer herself was four months pregnant. "You'd think you'd become more able to handle those difficult calls (because) you would've had the experience. You'd know how to protect yourself," she said, reflecting on a 32-year career. "But it's the opposite. Your life experience, maturity, empathy has grown and now you can associate with so many more calls."

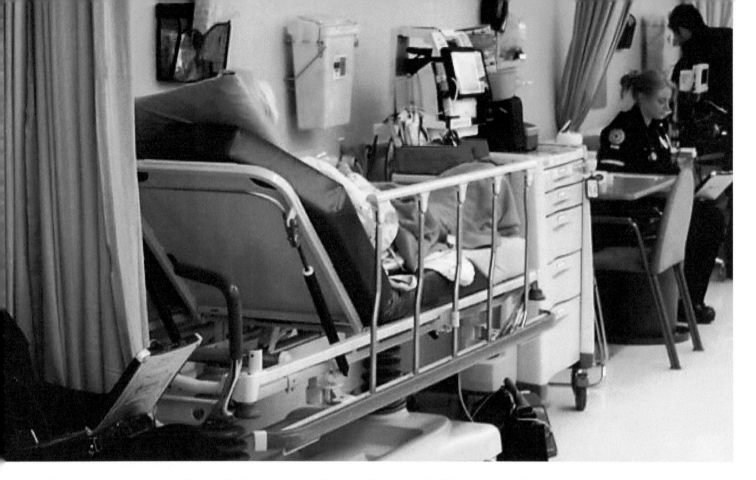

Patients in stretchers line a hallway at the Peter Lougheed Centre while they wait with paramedics for an emergency department bed space to open up. Paramedics continue to provide care while waiting with their patients. (Courtesy of AHS EMS Archives)

THE HALLWAY MEDIC

In the new millennium, EMS was becoming more a part of the health-care system, yet was still being funded out of the municipal budget. Alberta's municipalities lobbied for years for the province to take more responsibility for the cost. In 2005, the province gave a $55-million grant to municipalities to offset the cost, but it was a drop in the bucket. The cost of labour, population growth and an aging population were all putting pressure on the City's EMS budget.

At the same time, the job description of a paramedic was increasingly becoming that of a "hallway medic." The number of calls per crew on any given shift dropped dramatically due to paramedics needing to wait with their patients, treating them in hospital hallways until a bed and nurses became available. In the most drastic scenarios, a crew might be waiting in a hospital for the majority of their 12-hour shift. An emergency ward couldn't and wouldn't refuse a patient, and there were not enough long-term beds for patients, so the backups piled up. It was becoming more common to have a Code Red, meaning there were no ambulances available in the city because they were all on calls. By June 2006, Calgary had registered more Code Reds in the previous six months than in the past 20 years combined. Paramedics were stuck in hallways and on average, patients were waiting more than two hours for an emergency department bed in 2006/07, compared with 68 minutes four years earlier.[20]

"It was damaging to the system," said Tom Sampson. "It was like someone changed the job description of our paramedics without consulting them, management or the medical advisory committee. The protracted waits caused response times to not be as important anymore because you were coming late anyway. People said, 'I didn't sign up to be in the hallway, I signed up to go out and take care of the next badly injured patient...' To this day I don't believe that paramedics should have any place in the hallway. ... The only way an ambulance is valuable on the street is if it's there and not tied up in a hospital."

In 2004, the Alberta government had consolidated health care by condensing its 17 health regions into nine boards. In 2008, it went further, announcing it would centralize all health care under the umbrella of a new Alberta Health Services (AHS), a massive multi-billion-dollar provincial authority. It was intended to save money on the largest line item in the Alberta budget, while also standardizing health-care delivery across the province for the betterment of patients. And emergency medical services were going to be integrated into health care as part of AHS, to the surprise of many longtime paramedics.

Sampson had been pushing the province for more funding for years, concerned about hospital wait times and ambulance response times. "In some ways I feel that I was so vociferous about the hospital wait times that in some ways they took EMS out of the City because we protested too much about those hospital waits and the impact they were having on our patients. I feel it was a way of shutting us up," he said. Sampson said a Calgary Health Region Authority employee once told him,

---

20 Lang, Michelle. "Hospital Crisis Brewing for Years." *Calgary Herald*, Feb. 21, 2008. https://search.proquest.com/docview/243459056?accountid=46584.

VITAL SIGNS

"As long as the drinks are free at the bar, the bar can never be big enough."

"The analogy they were trying to give me was as long as you could walk into emerg unimpeded you could never have an emerg department big enough. ... It was just not good. It was no good for our patients and it wasn't good for our paramedics and EMTs."

THE PROVINCIAL HEALTH CARE ERA 2009-2019

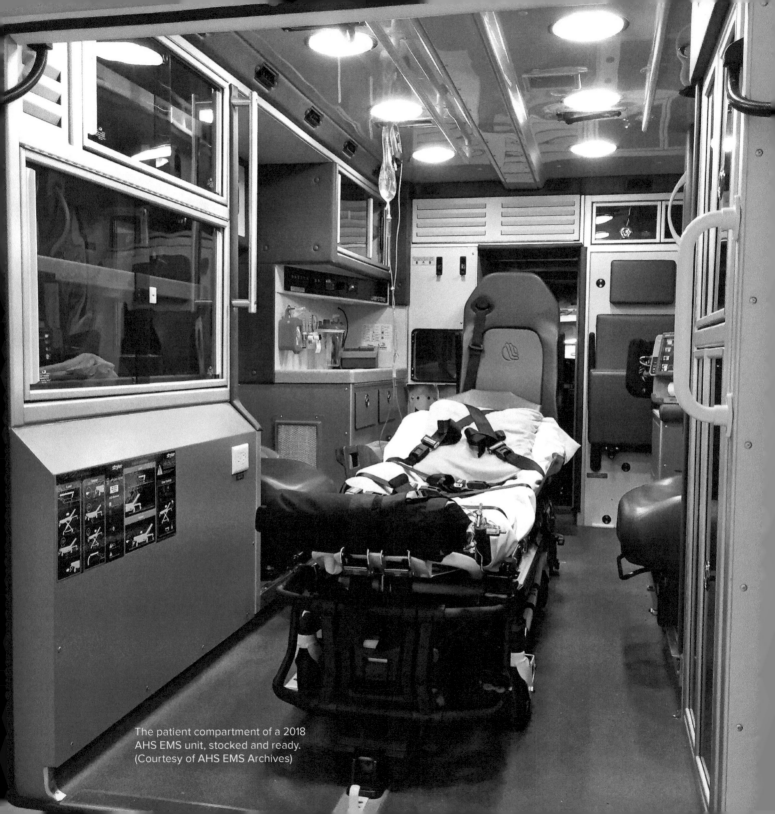
The patient compartment of a 2018 AHS EMS unit, stocked and ready. (Courtesy of AHS EMS Archives)

THE PROVINCIAL HEALTH CARE ERA 2009–2019

COMING TOGETHER IN A CRISIS

Creating the Alberta Health Services superboard was a massive undertaking, and bringing EMS into the big tent was one piece of a complex puzzle. Among many goals for the transition from more than 70 distinct ambulance services into one was for it to be seamless for patients across Alberta.

There was a lot of trepidation from Calgary staff in the lead-up to April 1, 2009. Some of those nervous feelings dissipated as it became more clear that the job would fundamentally be the same and would be done by the same people. But not everyone. This was the end of Tom Sampson's career as EMS chief.

"I felt like I was abandoning my staff and I felt like I was abandoning family members," said Sampson. Sampson and the City negotiated with AHS to make him part of the transition team for this massive change to the ambulance service. "I was very torn," he said. "But at the same time, it was very clear to me that Health wasn't prepared to financially keep what I was doing in place…Talk about rip your heart out."

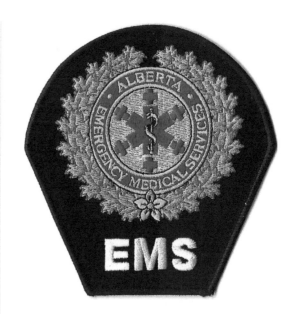

Shoulder crest of Alberta Health Services EMS, 2009–present. (Courtesy of AHS EMS Archives)

Sampson said he wonders whether his longtime leadership position was part of the reason they couldn't find an appropriate place for him in the new system. "Maybe I would represent too much of holding on to the past when they needed to move forward to a different model. Who knows. I don't know. I know in the end it was better for me even though I didn't think it at the time," he said.

Behind the scenes, the pace was frenetic leading up to transition day. In Calgary alone, AHS was taking over a fleet of around 80 EMS vehicles, plus hundreds of staff (and all their work history and vacation balances), plus lease agreements on City facilities that EMS operated out of, said Darren Sandbeck. Sandbeck led the EMS transition in Calgary on behalf of AHS. Now Chief Paramedic for AHS, Sandbeck said there wasn't a single blip in service over the transition, a point he's very proud of.

Consolidating dozens of ambulance services meant standardizing vehicles, equipment and medical protocols across the province. That, in theory, makes it a borderless system with consistently high-quality care.

While Albertans expect and assume that they'll get the same high quality of care when they call 911, no matter where in the province they are, that just wasn't the case prior to 2009. The borderless system also makes dispatch more efficient. For example, in 2008 say an ambulance from outside of Calgary had transported into the city and was on their way back home. If a 911 call came into Calgary for the highway they were travelling on, they wouldn't be dispatched even if they were the closest unit, because they weren't part of the system. Today, the province-wide dispatch system knows where every ambulance is and can send the closest unit.

One of the overarching goals of creating AHS was to help the health-care system run more efficiently and effectively in a province where the population had increased 20%, from 2.9 million in 2000 to 3.5 million by 2008. It was a hotbed of growth fuelled once again by a prosperous oil economy; Canada's population only increased by 8%, or about 2.5 million during the same time. The pressure on heath care was immense. In Calgary, the number of available hospital beds hadn't caught up with the aging, growing population, and was still feeling the effects of hospital closures a decade earlier. By the end of 2009, emergency department waiting times reached a crisis point. "Patients were now waiting an average of 14.4 hours before being admitted to hospital, 30 per cent longer than in 2007," when it was

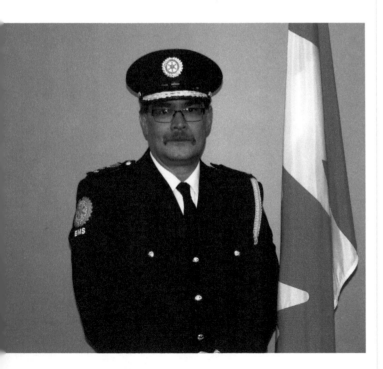

Darren Sandbeck, Chief Paramedic, AHS. (Courtesy of AHS EMS Archives)

THE PROVINCIAL HEALTH CARE ERA 2009–2019

11.1 hours.[21] Funding more long-term care beds, hospital beds, doctors and nurses may have been the solution. But building hospitals and hiring professionals takes time and money that the government didn't have—and perhaps wasn't ready to spend if they had. In 2008, a global economic recession hit Alberta right in the barrel and the sizeable health-care budget was again targeted for cutting, making significant change untenable.

Of course, illness and injury don't wait around for the ideal moment to strike. In 2009, Calgary's paramedics were fully braced for a pandemic flu to hit the city. H1N1, or swine flu, was a new version of the Spanish flu that killed an estimated 50 to 100 million people in 1918. H1N1 tended to hit younger, healthy populations harder than the seasonal flu. AHS braced for impact with specialized paramedic response units and flu response units. These were single paramedic units equipped with equipment specifically for H1N1 cases. When a suspected case was called in, these flu response units were prepared for the scene, limiting their possible contact with the virus. They would make a decision on whether a patient needed to be transported to the hospital—were they sick enough to warrant a hospital visit when it also meant potentially allowing the virus to spread?

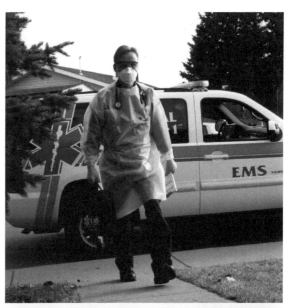

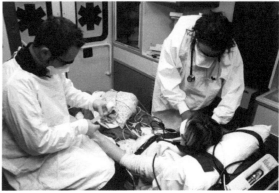

H1N1 training. (Courtesy of AHS EMS Archives)

---

21 McClure, Matt. "Doctors Say ER Crisis Warnings Fell on Deaf Ears; Tories 'Didn't Get' Urgency of Increasing Wait Times." *Calgary Herald*, Dec 5, 2010. https://search.proquest.com/docview/816361320?accountid=46584.

VITAL SIGNS

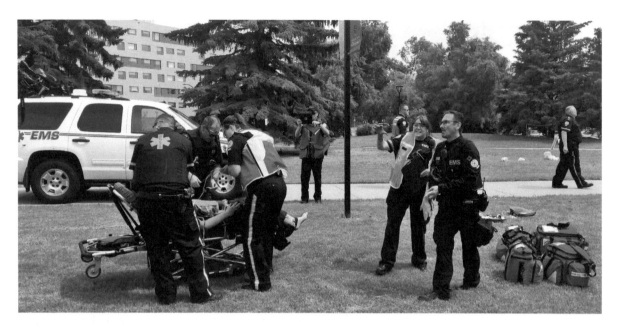

An MCI training scenario, June 2017. (Courtesy of AHS EMS Archives)

The special units also minimized contact for paramedics, because losing a significant amount of staff would put even more pressure on the system. Despite the fears of how deadly H1N1 might be, a report into the flu response found that 64 individuals died as a direct result of the virus, the third-highest mortality rate for flu season since 1983.[22]

---

22 Government of Alberta. Review of Deaths Occurring In Alberta During the 2009 Influenza Pandemic. Edmonton: Government of Alberta, 2012.

EMS has response plans in case of Mass Casualty Incidents, or MCIs. The name is a bit deceiving as these plans are used in cases where there may be zero patients. For example, if a nursing home were being evacuated due to a fire, an MCI plan would be used even if nobody was hurt. It's about being proactive. An MCI plan was used in 2000 at Pine Lake, AB, when a tornado touched down, causing chaos, injuries in large numbers of patients and deaths. There were also MCIs in place during the 2013 floods in Calgary and High River, when the overflowing rivers caused an estimated $5 billion in damage and claimed five lives.

Sometimes a MCI plan is about transporting the disaster from the scene to a hospital. A scene with 20 patients who need to go to the hospital isn't typical, so there needs to be a system in place to allocate them appropriately by triaging at the scene. It answers the question "How do we provide structure and order to a chaotic scene?" and can be enacted whenever anything happens that will or has already overwhelmed normal EMS resources.

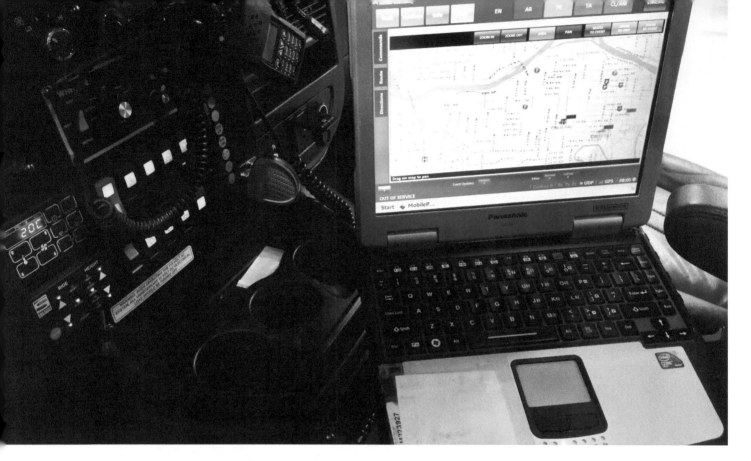

An AHS paramedic's mobile office is now fully digital. (Courtesy of AHS EMS Archives)

THE NEW DAY JOB

After the initial transition to AHS, the day-to-day job of a Calgary paramedic saw some changes, too. Crews had already switched from paper patient care reports to digital in 2008 and more digitization was on the way. The computerized dispatch system uses GPS to track ambulances and send them to calls based on their location. It "was like the land of technology," said Terri Nixon, a paramedic who trained in Toronto before joining the department in Calgary in 2008. She'd been used to the paper maps she used in Toronto ("It was the same map book you'd get at Walmart.") and found her early days navigating an ambulance in Toronto frustrating and stressful—especially when it was an 0400 hours cardiac call. "Coming from a different service, Calgary is much better than what I was coming from. Some people here don't know how good they've got it because they haven't worked anywhere else," she said.

In 2018/19, the Alberta Health Services budget is $15.2 billion, and the government is constantly looking for ways to use provincial health resources effectively and efficiently and take some pressure off the system. One of those approaches is community paramedics, who attend to patients in their homes when a doctor's office visit or hospital stay is either difficult or unnecessary. Their patients are typically people who, without continual, reliable medical follow-up might find themselves back in the health-care system instead of being able to live in their home. Community paramedics provide assessment, treatment and follow-up, and can help teach patients or their loved ones what's necessary to keep them in good health. Community paramedics don't work on ambulances; it's a distinct role. Their day-to-day is a blend between a street medic and a home care nurse and they're increasingly important in Alberta's health-care landscape.

Paramedic Daphne Stevenson, like many of her predecessors, found her way to the profession in part under the influence of watching the William Shatner-hosted *Rescue 911* as a kid—and a love of driving fast. Stevenson said she knows that she and her EMS colleagues make a difference for people every day, but there's one type of call that, for her, has particular impact: a palliative care call.

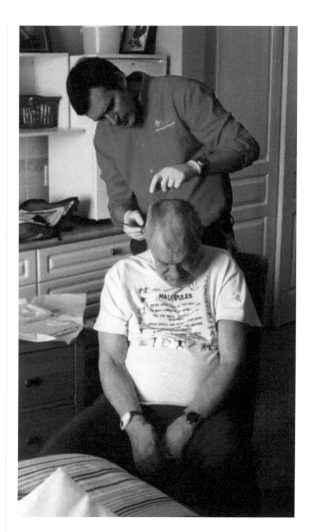

A community paramedic cares for a patient in their home, helping them stay in their home and cut down on additional strain on the medical system. (Courtesy of AHS EMS Archives)

Stevenson has attended to more palliative patients in recent years than most of her fellow paramedics. She said every time it's a mix of heartbreak and gratitude that she could help a family at a loved one's end of life. "When someone wishes to die at home in the comfort of their home, with their family there to help them do that with dignity—to help keep their last wishes is one of the most important things that we do," said Stevenson. In some cases, she administers medication to ease pain in the final days or weeks of a person's life. Other times, she's there with a family in a loved one's last hour. Notably, this end-of-life care isn't related to physician-assisted death. It's "incredibly hard" to be part of a family's grief, but at the same time, she said she knows that years from now, when a child has grown up and can look back at the help EMS gave their dying parent, they'll appreciate those moments and will respect the profession.

The wide range of emergencies today still includes things like a young person dealing with their first hangover or a person who cut their fingernails too short. Terri Nixon said she sometimes has to stop and appreciate that so many of the things she does almost by rote every day are things her patients will remember for their entire lives. She once helped a patient who, intending to prepare for her first Rocky Mountain hike, tested a canister of bear spray in her kitchen. After neighbours called 911 and brought the woman into their home, Nixon attended and was, within moments, washing and rinsing the naked woman in the neighbour's shower to get the burning bear spray off her skin. It was a painful 30 minutes of showering for the woman, but by the end, she was laughing and said to Nixon, "I'm never going to forget you. You're part of the most embarrassing thing I've ever done."

Stevenson said she and her colleagues still spend too much time waiting in hospital hallways with patients. And she deals with the occasional patient who has called 911 for help getting up from a fall and doesn't believe "two ladies" are going to be able to help him up off the floor. She relishes the challenge.

Paramedic Ashley McKay said she worries that EMS is too short on resources these days due to hallway waits. It means there are few ambulances on the street available for other calls. "We're all waiting for that big event to happen," she said. "How we would be able to attend that call appropriately is really scary. That would take so many resources off the street." McKay recalled a recent New Year's Eve when she was on the last ambulance available in the city. She responded to a call halfway across the city for someone reporting chest pain. By the time they got there, they learned the patient was playing a board game with his family, laughing harder than he had ever laughed in his life, and that, rather than a cardiac incident, was causing the chest pain. McKay wonders if that non-emergency could have been dealt with by dispatch rather than taking the last ambulance off the street.

"I think part of the challenge is the whole health-care system is challenged right now," said Tom Sampson, now looking from the outside in. "They've been dealing in crisis for so long, it's not a crisis anymore, it's just (business as usual). ... In some ways I'm glad that I don't have to try and solve all of the health challenges for them. I think that you could take out the top 10 people and put 10 more people in of your picking and within a year you'd feel the same way about that because the system is so difficult to fix.

"What I can tell you is that paramedics are a big part of the solution. They always have been and always will be."

In the midst of that frustration, McKay noted how important paramedics are in filling a need in the health-care system. "We're more than just individuals in blue with tubes and IVs coming to save your life," she said. "We're so much more." In five years in the career, she's played the role of taxi driver, babysitter, social worker, psychologist and shoulder to cry on for people having the worst days of their lives. It takes its toll, she said. "We're destroyed inside and expected to go to the next call… and be 100%. It's not possible."

For retired paramedic Carolyn Kremer, unpredictability was part of the draw to the job. She said she appreciated the autonomy of working within protocols and performing under tough circumstances. Kremer said that anyone who wants a long career as a paramedic today will have to stay away from the political side. "You have to keep it in your own sandbox," she said. "If you're trying to look after all the politics and all the issues of hospital waits and lack of whatever, you're not going to make it. … Just do what you're there to do. Don't try to change the system."

After decades as a paramedic, Claude Belobersycky had taken some time off the job and was contemplating a more permanent career change in the final years of the City of Calgary era. Then, a totally unexpected moment made the decision for him. He and his wife were driving Country Hills Boulevard when a van veered in front of them and flipped over. They, along with other drivers who witnessed it, pulled over to try to help. Belobersycky and three or four others helped flip the van back up onto its wheels. Belobersycky had been off the job for months, but leapt into action. The driver wasn't breathing, had no pulse and his head was wedged between the vehicle console and steering wheel. While Belobersycky questioned what he could possibly do with no equipment, he jumped into the back of the van and held the driver's neck secure, doing his best while suspecting a neck injury. A man came up to offer help and it turned out he was a director of respiratory health. Belobersycky told him he was just the man he needed because his patient wasn't breathing and he may have a broken neck. Belobersycky said he thought he'd need to perform a cricothyrotomy—make an incision to open the airway—with the knife

VITAL SIGNS

he carried in his back pocket. The respiratory director was wide-eyed but fished the knife out for Belobersycky. And just as the off-duty paramedic was about to make an incision, the fire department arrived and was able to use a bag valve mask to revive the driver in seconds. The incident made it crystal clear to Belobersycky that he was in the right career. "Every day when you get up you start thinking, 'I wonder what's going to happen today,'" he said. "It causes a bit of angst but it's kind of exciting because you never know." Belobersycky worked for another 12 years, retiring after 44 years on the job.

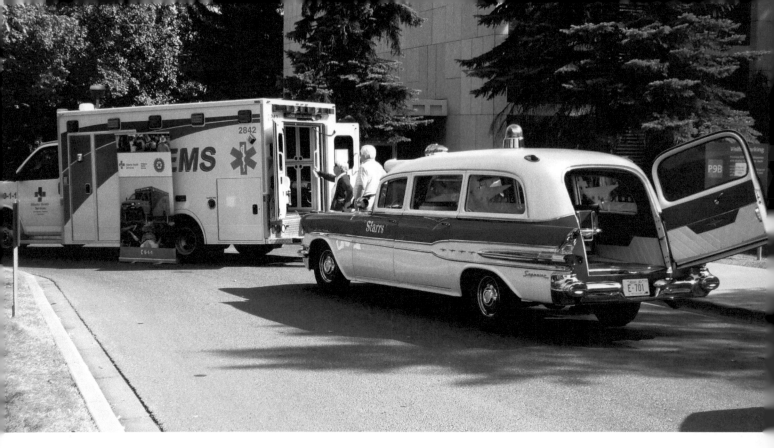

At the 40th anniversary of the Paramedic Training Program at SAIT in 2012, guests could see at a glance just how much has changed. (Courtesy of Tim Prieur)

THEN AND NOW

For those who have worked through multiple eras in Calgary's EMS history, it's hard not to make comparisons through the years. That hindsight makes for a greater appreciation of the years of the past—but also a lot of gratitude for medical and technological advancements that have helped practitioners and patients alike.

Gino Savoia, who has lived more than 40 years of Calgary's EMS history, and is now a clinical educator for AHS, sees both challenges and opportunities for EMS today.

"The biggest challenge for us in Calgary, is that we went from a relatively small autonomous group where decisions could be made extremely quickly to a provincial model where it's suddenly an elephant," Savoia said. "To turn or stop an elephant takes forever." While the City department could implement new protocols or procedures within hours, today there are more levels of approval and consultation. In many cases, changes need to be executable across the province before they can be executed anywhere. In such a large organization, a switch-up in medication or equipment may not always be communicated all the way down the line. For example, a nausea drug for kids in liquid form was replaced on ambulances with a pill that was double the dose. When staff needed the drug and couldn't find the liquid form, they thought it had been used up and not replaced. When they did find the pill, they didn't have a pill cutter on hand to get the proper dose. To make this discovery in front of a patient is "a very big deal," said Savoia, and frustrating for field staff.

Finding time to train medics has always been tough and still is today. Calgary had long had field trainers who were able to train by attending calls and acting as checks and balances for medics. They could help on scene or identify when additional training in a specific area was required. The field trainer model has been replaced by AHS EMS with a clinical educator model, where educators lecture more broadly to practitioners across the province. It's expensive to pull medics off of active duty and cover their positions for training. Savoia said Calgary EMS staff today only get about 10 hours of mandatory training annually, and

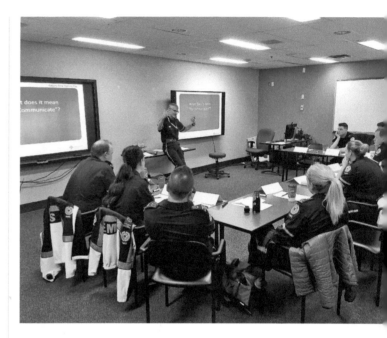

Clinical educator CPR training. (Courtesy of AHS EMS Archives)

most of that training is for recertification of certain skills, such as CPR. And there's no guarantee of even that if they get called back to the street on training day.

At the same time, being part of an organization with deep pockets has major benefits. The province invested in power cots for all ambulances, spending about $50,000 per ambulance on the hydraulic stretchers for the $25-million project. Saving medics from lifting patients—a significant cause of injuries in the profession—is a big deal. Savoia said "there's no way" the City department would have been able to undertake that scale of a project in a one-year timeframe. The provincial fleet is phenomenal, first-class and consistent. (Not all tech and equipment improvements are universally appreciated, though. Some staff have nicknamed their computer-aided dispatch units in ambulances "SkyNet" after the sinister computer system from the *Terminator* movie franchise that aims to eliminate all humans. The mapping software sends ambulance crews to calls based on its own algorithms—which are sometimes vastly different to what paramedics feel is the best route.)

Being part of the provincial health-care system in a formalized way allows paramedics to follow up on their patients after the fact. Trying to do that in the old days "was like pulling teeth. If you were successful it took months," said Savoia. Follow-up is key to paramedics finding out if they made the right decisions and treatment. That curiosity allows them to become better at what they do. "Coming from a different service, Calgary is much better than what I was coming from," said Terri Nixon, referring to her early career in the Toronto area. She said that from high-quality equipment to the specialty teams paramedics can train to work in, and jobs for Advanced Care Paramedics, there are broader options for the career here than elsewhere in Canada.

Claude Belobersycky retired from AHS in 2017. He said that being part of the health-care system has facilitated more trust in paramedics. "They've enabled us now to make those critical, gut moment, split-second decisions on our own," he said. "Yes, you have a protocol… but not every call is cookie cutter like that. Sometimes there's like three or four different things going on at the same time and you have to almost play detective and think outside the box and then you have to make a decision." He said that independence and trust is good pressure to ensure paramedics keep up their skill level.

Acting as one tiny cog in a massive organization, which employs more Albertans than any other, can be tough. Naturally, as the city has grown, the tight-knit group of EMS staff has grown. Now, with about 1,000 people working in EMS in the Calgary Zone (which includes areas surrounding the city) that community feel has changed. There's a limit to the level of trust that can be built not just within EMS, but also with emergency department nurses and doctors in such a large community.

Dr. Peter Gant said he used to be able to develop close relationships with medics, taking 20 or 30 minutes to discuss a patient and work together to treat them at the hospital. Where possible, Gant would provide oversight while directing the paramedic to perform a procedure, such as intubating a patient. It was a chance to review the medic's skills and for the medic to do so in a safe environment.

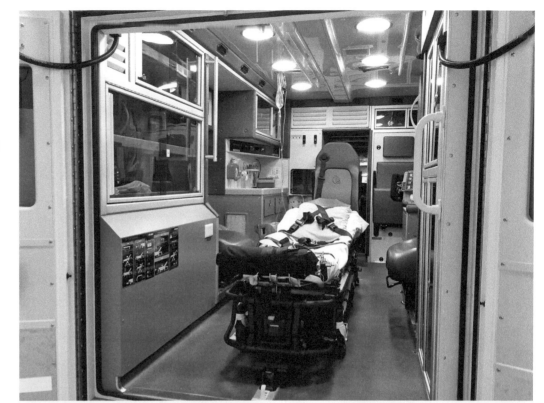

The EMS Foundation sponsored the initial trial of a power cot system for AHS ambulances, which was subsequently adopted province-wide. These stretchers can move in and out of the ambulance at the touch of a button. (Courtesy of AHS EMS Archives)

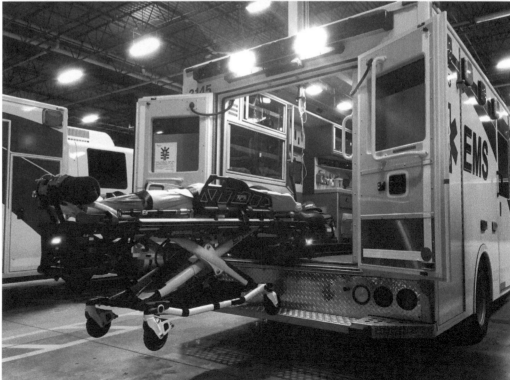

"I always felt it was a tremendous communication and learning experience for the providers," he said. "We (emergency physicians) have disconnected ourselves from EMS in a bad way."

Today, Alberta's paramedics require liability insurance. It's a reflection both of their increased scope of practice and independence. "You're the guy," said Belobersycky. "That's created a whole new level of responsibility, which I think is good because it kind of forces people who are paramedics to take the initiative to understand and make sure they know their discipline inside and out."

EMS in Calgary has long provided public safety services alongside medical. That piece of their identity is somewhat outside the purview of AHS and has taken a backseat to health care. Nobody else in Alberta's health-care system works so independently and in such potentially hazardous conditions as paramedics. Savoia noted that, following up on a Health and Wellness initiative, AHS provided a one-time self-defense course to paramedics after a very public incident of two paramedics being assaulted on the job. However, it wasn't made part of ongoing training and recertification. Savoia said it's an excellent initiative, but he doubts whether it can make a significant difference in the long term.

Tom Sampson, who is now firmly in the public safety realm as chief of Calgary's Emergency Management Agency, said the public sees paramedics as part of public safety, like police officers. "You can't just be a medic capable of inserting IVs. You have to be able to crawl in the back of a car and you have to be able to scramble down the side of a hill. There's some public safety pieces that go into everybody's work."

A typical tour for a Calgary paramedic is as busy as it's ever been. "We constantly don't have enough ambulances in the city," said Daphne Stevenson, noting there was a time when paramedics could sleep most of the way through some night shifts. But all the same, "going to work is awesome," she said, praising her colleagues and patients alike. It's medicine meets customer service. Stevenson said she loves meeting new people and hearing their stories, even when someone has called 911 more for the company than what some people might consider an emergency. "You think you'd see the worst in people, but you don't," she said. "When people are at their worst or their most stressed-out, that's when they're their truest selves. And that's their kindest."

She recounted one call where an elderly man had suffered a cardiac incident and despite her work, Stevenson was unable to save his life. When Stevenson faced the heartbreaking moment of telling the man's wife of 50 years that he had died, the woman thanked her for trying and offered to make her a cup of tea. Fellow paramedic Nixon said she didn't expect, when she started her paramedic education 12 years ago, that there would be so many deep, if fleeting, human connections in her career. "You walk into somebody's house, somebody's life and very briefly you're completely part of them," she said. "They tell their deepest, darkest secrets. They don't hold anything back.

"People call paramedics when they don't know what to do," Nixon said. "At the moment when they've completely lost control, that's when they call 911."

NEVER FORGOTTEN

VITAL SIGNS

TIMELINE OF CALGARY AMBULANCE SERVICES
(Courtesy of Peter Adsten)

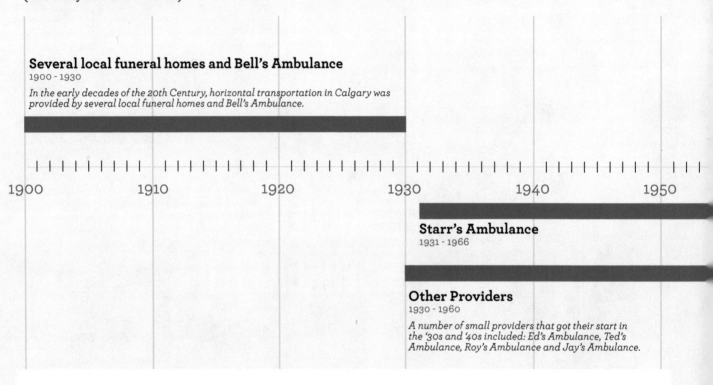

Several local funeral homes and Bell's Ambulance
1900 - 1930

In the early decades of the 20th Century, horizontal transportation in Calgary was provided by several local funeral homes and Bell's Ambulance.

Starr's Ambulance
1931 - 1966

Other Providers
1930 - 1960

A number of small providers that got their start in the '30s and '40s included: Ed's Ambulance, Ted's Ambulance, Roy's Ambulance and Jay's Ambulance.

This is just one version of the history of pre-hospital care in Calgary. It's one written thanks to the thoughtful recollections—not to mention their collections—of many of the people who lived it.

NEVER FORGOTTEN

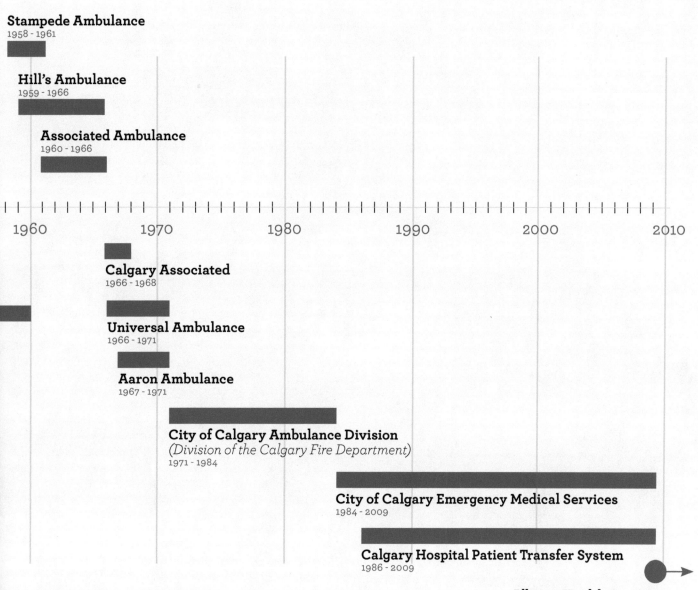

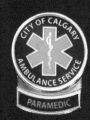 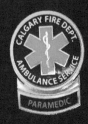 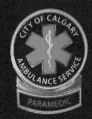 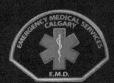
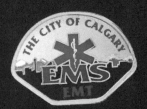 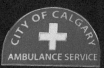 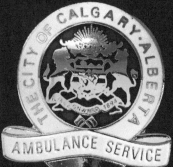 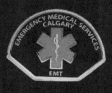 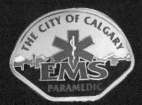
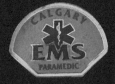 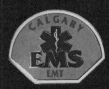 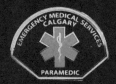

Shoulder crest pin set created to mark the transition of EMS services from the City of Calgary to the province, 2009. (Courtesy of AHS EMS Archives)

A FINAL THOUGHT, THOUGH NEVER THE FINAL WORD

The last half-century has seen tremendous advancements in the field of medicine. This is particularly apparent in the area of pre-hospital emergency medical care. In Calgary alone, over the course of even a single medic's career, we've seen multiple eras. From the days of driving fast and applying the sticky side of the bandage down, to making split-second decisions to save lives in the most unforgiving circumstances.

The stories captured in these pages are just a fraction of the history of EMS delivery in Calgary, but it's hoped they weave a clear picture of the roots, triumphs and challenges of the "ambulance people." It is dedicated to those men and women who have devoted their lives to the care of others, and to future generations who will carry the torch forward another 50 years.

This is just one version of the history of pre-hospital care in Calgary. It's one written thanks to the thoughtful recollections—not to mention their collections—of many of the people who lived it.

Thank you to Bill McComb, whose archives, memories and generosity of time were a particular asset from outlining to final reading of this book. Gary Fisher, for sharing so many tales of the early days of this history. Paul Morck for filling in gaps along the way, and reviewing early drafts and making this writer laugh. Tom Sampson, despite what your wife says, you're a fine historian! Gino Savoia for sharing decades of history with us and for reviewing the manuscript.

A massive dose of gratitude is due to everyone who contributed to this historical journey: Ron McManus, Ann and Richard Sigurdson, Darren Sandbeck, Mike Plato, Stuart Brideaux, Doug Odney, Brian Boechler, Ron Firth, Dave Jensen, Brent Thorkelson, Daphne Stevenson, Terri Nixon, Ashley McKay, Carolyn Kremer, Dr. Gil Curry, Dr. Peter Gant, Bob "Bullet" Willis and Claude Belobersycky. A special thanks also to Dell Harrison, Jared Hendry, Jennifer Van Der Straeten and Lara Surring, who offered their support at the first EMS Foundation Gala in May 2018.

And particular recognition must go to Dr. Tim Prieur of the EMS Foundation, who believed in this history project from the outset and ensured all of its many pieces would come together so the world could read it and so that these stories would be remembered.

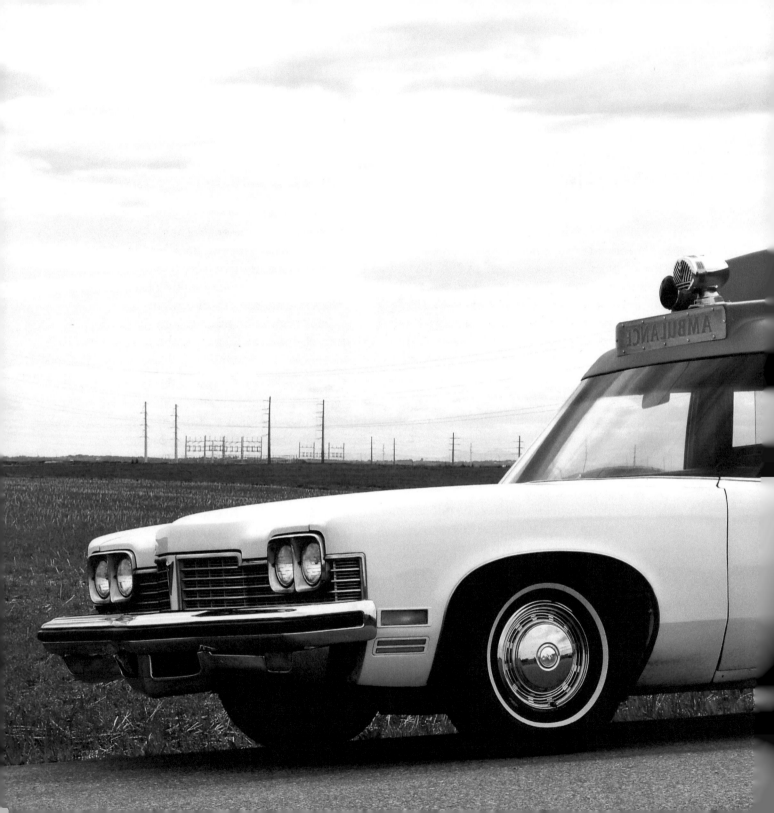

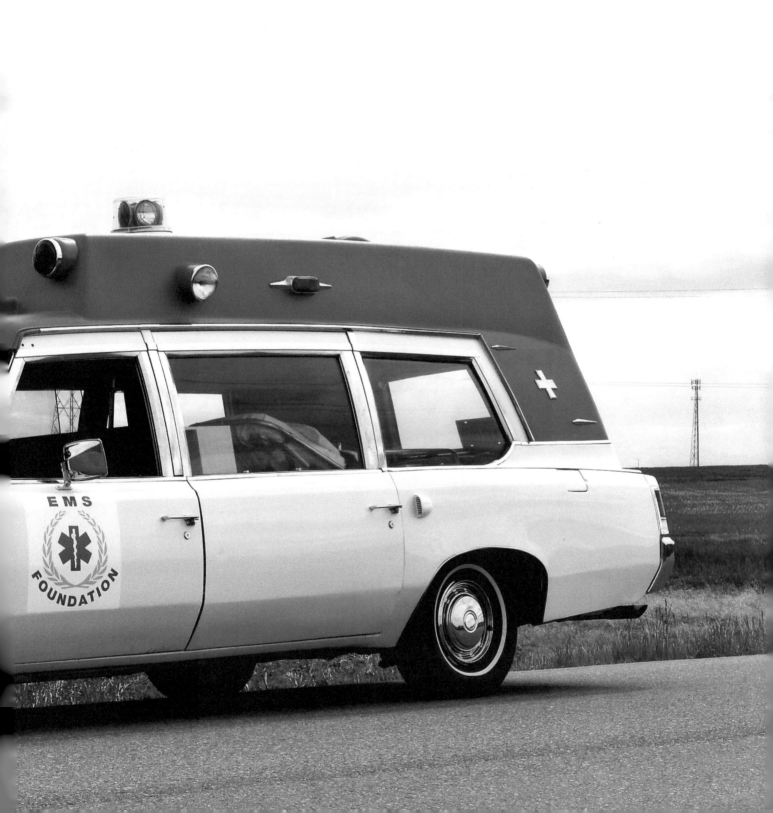

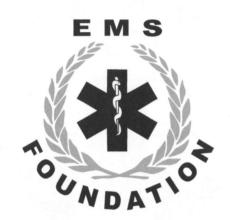

CPSIA information can be obtained
at www.ICGtesting.com
Printed in the USA
LVHW020348140519
617705LV00001B/1/P